To Wendy

Introduction

What's the use of an autopsy? What's it like to be flight-phobic, agoraphobic, terrified of public speaking or extremely shy? What hidden damages can car accidents inflict? What's it like to survive the Nazi concentration camps? What is chronic pain? What is exposure therapy? How does one prove that a drug really works? My path of learning about these diverse subjects took me from one continent to another, from one medical specialty to another, from one research project to another and finally to the Courts of Law.

I am describing anxiety, pain, trauma and how they can be understood, but without recommending any particular treatment. What's appropriate now will change and continue to change. Instead I am describing how observations must be assembled carefully, completely and without preconceived notion to be useful, in medicine and in other walks of life.

I am leaving out most things personal unless they illustrate a particular point. I am also leaving out a lot of people who I love and care for because they did not change my work.

Last but not least, any writing about medicine needs a disclaimer. I'll give you two.

- This is not a self-help book. I am merely telling a story. Ask your doctor or lawyer if you want help.
- I write this from memory after fourteen years of retirement. And even I make the occasional mistake (according to my spouse).

1. How It All Started

According to an old German tale all babies wait in a pond called the *Kinderteich* (babies' pond). They splash about until the stork arrives, bundles them up and delivers them to a random destination where overjoyed parents await. Actual procreation may look different, but the *Kinderteich* is accurate in another way. It's a nice illustration of the lottery of birth and something I will get back to later. The stork chose Southern Germany for me and deposited my bundle smack into the middle of WWII. My parents were doctors in a small town by the name of Schwaebisch Hall. Both worked at the *Diakonissenanstalt*, a large hospital known locally as *the Diak.* A Protestant order ran it. Its grounds included a farm, residences for the sisters of the order, a small nursing home for ailing retirees and residences for staff. A few mentally handicapped persons also lived there in a protected work arrangement. We lived in a converted ward right in the hospital. My mother worked in pediatrics, my dad in internal medicine and radiology. Most of the time he was at the Russian front. I wet his knee when we first met. He shouldn't have put me there.

Fast-forward to the year of 1945. Picture the time when the Nazi regime was collapsing around everybody's ears. The window of our dining room faced west, a fact of some significance as allied bombers approached from there. We were having lunch. I sat at the side of the table that faced the window, placed perfectly for an early warning system. A large formation of planes approached from the West with an increasing roar. I was transfixed by the sight and pointed at it. My interest was not shared in the expected manner. Instead of lunch plus entertainment, somebody whisked me away and down into the bowels of the hospital. A deafening crash shook everything. A bomb had hit us. The reason for the commotion was a military airport located on a plain just above the hospital. German Messerschmitt 262 jet fighters were based there and Allied Bomber Command had become interested. Lots of bomb craters throughout town and near the railway station bore further witness to their efforts. A few days later a nurse took me outside for some fresh air during a lull in the fighting. Loud bangs and the stutter of machine guns chased us back inside. On another occasion my dad lifted me up for a look from our kitchen window. It overlooked the river valley below and a village we had visited days before. A bomb had hit a house there. It was ablaze like a huge torch. I liked it. He took me to a crater a few hundred yards from the hospital where plane had crashed into the hillside during a bombing run. I liked that too. My parents were with me and nothing bad could happen. After the fighting was all over dad put me into a small plane that had crash-landed near the airport. He lifted me into the cockpit and I played with the controls.

From my vantage point war was hugely interesting.

Losing my mother soon after at the tender age of four changed this happy frame of mind. A stepmother entered my life after her death and replaced warmth with rough treatment. I hid in a closet when the going got rough. Seven decades later mothballs still smell reassuring. When dad caught her at it, he was blunt in my defense and it didn't happen again. Still my hackles rise when someone enjoys the exercise of power a little bit too much.

We lived at the hospital for six more years after the war. I had the run of the place. A hundred nurses mothered me. I "helped" in the hospital kitchen, stirred soups in enormous electrical kettles from the top of a stool and developed advanced skills as a food taster. A visit to the septic laundry resulted in a scrub-down, a second one into the operating room during surgery in a caution and a third to the morgue in an encounter with a dead motorcyclist. A maid upped the ante on the last one. The motorcyclist might have been a "non-dead," she said. He might be ready and waiting to sit up suddenly in his coffin to do nasty things. I swallowed this tale hook, line and sinker and got really scared of dead bodies, not what you want for a medical career. But I built a solid base for one in other ways.

We lived just a few floors below the radiology department. My dad looked like an alien in the morning with his dark-red goggles that he wore to preserve night vision. The equipment of the day produced only faint images that had to be viewed in the dark. He also put on a heavy lead apron against radiation. I joined him behind the screen, equally protected. His patients didn't seem to mind the child radiologist. And a gastric ulcer is a small sensation when demonstrated on a screen by a barium swallow.

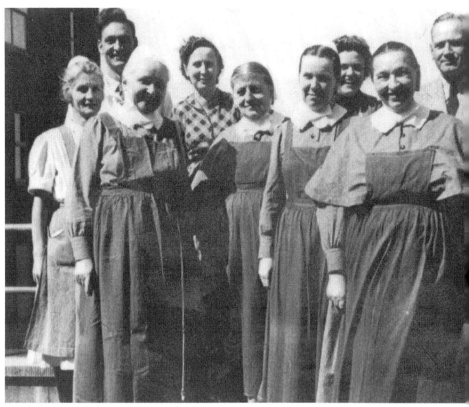

Dad (top right) and his radiology crew

After the War doctors were in short supply. My dad moonlighted in family practice. I accompanied him for a home visit in the countryside to a man with ascites, the fluid that accumulates in the abdomen in liver failure. We came to a dismal-looking little house. His patient was in bed in a cold room. Dad lit the wood stove and waited for the room to warm, then drained the ascites into a bucket through a large-bore needle. There was no question of payment on this occasion. Other home visits were more remunerative. Large farms were the best. They paid with eggs, milk, hunks of pork and poultry, sometimes with a hot meal. This went both ways. Dad was the farmers' source of health care and they were a source of food for us. One provided Christmas turkeys for years after we moved from the hospital into town. The turkeys wouldn't fit into our oven and the nuns roasted the beasts in the hospital kitchen. My job was to balance the casserole on the back seat of the car while making sure that the turkey tasted ok.

My old man also had some classy connections. One was a count that lived in a 16th century castle with surrounding moat and large grounds. His son was about my age. He took me to the stables and through stately rooms. I got to touch the famous "Iron Hand" from the Sixteen-hundreds, a prosthetic device used by an ancestor after his forearm had been chopped off in battle. Riding a scooter with balloon tires was another treat. It gave me a lasting taste for the life of the other half.

But it was the pig that really took the biscuit.

Food was rationed after the War. All live pigs were registered. None could be slaughtered without a permit. But, as always, there was a loophole. The pigs were registered but not their size. When a sow had piglets the black-market was on and my old man was in on it (and happy to fill me in on the details later). We set out in his car, a black two-stroke pre-War vintage DKW (*Deutscher Kraftwagen*) the occupying "*Amis*" (Americans) allowed him for his medical practice. Only this time we weren't visiting a sickbed. Instead we went to a farm and traded a piglet for a full-size pig. It was uncooperative at first and squealed when stuffed into the back of the car. But it kept quiet under a blanket while the engine was running. On the way home we came to an American roadblock. Dad stopped and kept the engine running. The soldiers knew him and waved us through. Once back at the hospital he got a pistol from a hiding place behind a high-voltage warning sign in the radiology unit and shot the pig. The night was spent butchering, frying, bottling and storing all the bits and pieces, this after everyone within smelling range had been bribed to keep mum.

Grammar school (*Volksschule*) was survival training. We also learned the basics of reading, writing and math. Teachers pulled hair and ears to improve attention spans. You got hit with a bamboo cane on your palm or fingers if you were bad. This was a called a "paw" and stung badly. If you were really bad, you were scheduled for a more thorough caning. Two boys assisted the teacher by pulling the perpetrator across their desk to expose his derriere. Everybody had to watch for the sake of betterment. Wise guys wore *Lederhosen* stuffed with newspaper for protection, or it was red welts and your parents would know. You yelped convincingly, even when well protected. American Quakers donated school lunches, stodgy soups that were brewed up locally and ladled into dented pots that did second duty as footballs. They tasted awful. Fridays brought relief with chocolate milk and soft buns. Religion was an important part of the curriculum. My hometown had played a prominent role during the Reformation. All my friends were Protestant. Logically, I attended Protestant instruction. However my family was Catholic. After some weeks or months my Lutheran fervor alerted them. They enquired and had me shifted to their side.

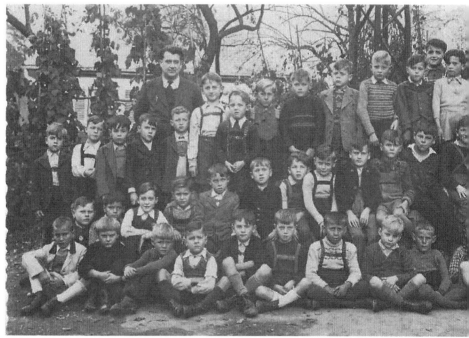

Grammar school; the author is the last one on the left, second row up, next to a future Lufthansa flight engineer.

Gymnasium (high school) was very different. It was highbrow, secular, and taught humanitarian ideals. Latin was taught from day one and for the entire nine years of the curriculum. We became closely acquainted with Greek gods and Roman emperors. Music lessons began with Johann Sebastian Bach, then moved to Mozart and Beethoven and stayed there. We sang Latin choral, me off-tune to get out of choral duty. Pop was frowned upon. Humanism was king and philosophy an integral part of the curriculum. We studied Kant, Humboldt and I read Nietzsche after an introduction by my dad. (Don't ask for quotes.) The natural sciences were mandatory. English and French were taught towards the end of the 9-year curriculum but not to a level that enabled conversation.

After graduation a school psychologist performed aptitude testing and recommended that I study Law. To see what it was like I sat in during a court hearing in Fuessen in Southern Bavaria. *Neuschwanstein* castle of King Ludwig fame dominated the scenery, standing out across the river valley against a mountainous backdrop. My uncle served as expert witness in a case about sausage casings. He was a crusty veterinarian with a red moustache who loved practical jokes and always wore the local get-up of green Loden cloth and *Haferl* shoes. Proceedings were in Bavarian. Northerners would have needed subtitles. My uncle's job was telling fake gut from the real thing and why the latter was better. I loved the setting but not the drawn-out proceedings and ignored the psychologist's advice. Later fate took me to the courts anyway.

I had been set on studying medicine since childhood and planned to open a practice in my hometown. I was going to lead a rural life as I had with my dad and uncle, go to the local pub and the *Stammtisch* (the locals' traditional table) where you can solve all the problems that politicians can't hack. It was a natural choice. I certainly had no plans to specialize in psychiatry. Even further from my mind was working on "funny farms," the large psychiatric institutions that sheltered the incurably insane until antipsychotic medications rendered them obsolete. But why not have a look? One day a visit to one near Lake Konstanz was on my dad's agenda and I went along. We set out in his gray Mercedes Benz, he in his gray suit, white shirt and gray tie. He was visiting his legal ward, a woman doctor who had been declared incompetent for reason of insanity. The landscape around Lake Konstanz is gorgeous, with mature woods, rolling hills, vineyards and small winding roads. The asylum was a grand old house in a park-like setting. Dad went inside to meet his ward. She accompanied him outside as he was leaving and he introduced us. She was painfully shy and barely looked me in the eye. She became tearful saying goodbye and dad promised another visit soon. A determination of "insanity" was open-ended then and there was nothing he could do to change her status.

Medical school

Entry to German medical training required a few months' work as a hospital orderly, to weed out the faint and nauseous. I served my time at the *Diak*, the place where I was born and had lived for the first ten years of my life. My mother had died there and dad would die there the year before my graduation. "Brother Kuch" was my handle. Brother Kuch did not get a special deal. At 6 a.m. sharpish he layered three aprons carefully over each other on top of a long monkish gown and proceeded to empty bedpans and urine flasks, then cleaned the lot. He wiped bums, made beds, collected greenish gobs of sputum for the lab and distributed chamomile tea down a linoleum-faced hallway. (I still abhor the smell of chamomile and the sight of linoleum.) Afterwards he sat down at a long table together with the other orderlies, said Grace and demolished a sustaining breakfast of pork cutlets, fried sausages, potatoes and more chamomile tea. Then the time might come to pick up an "*exitus*" (a "stiff" or dead body). The routine was to arrive when nobody was looking. The corpse was usually in a dark room, with curtains drawn and spookily quiet. The pair of orderlies who had drawn the short straw would lift it onto a covered gurney, wheel it to the elevator and out onto the street for the short run to the morgue, a small bungalow-shaped building shaded by large trees. We covered the distance in a hurry and rarely encountered anyone. A gallows' humor prevailed amongst orderlies and patients alike. Patients consoled us when the ghastly task came due, despite the fact that they too might occupy similar transport. One, a kindly innkeeper with an ailing liver, had a supply of schnapps hidden in his locker. He offered it around before and again after the deed was done.

Most patients were local farmers, hearty but gruff and not overly clean. We scrubbed new admissions until they glistened. According to a standing joke both feet needed cleaning, not just the afflicted one. After a week or two on the ward many also needed "emptying out". The hospital diet was high on starch and fat but low on fiber. Immobility did the rest. Requests for laxatives were routine, enemas a sought-after remedy. An old hand in these matters introduced Brother Kuch to a concoction that was easy to administer and fabulously effective. It contained warm glycerin, a pinch of salt and a secret ingredient for added potency. Once injected into the victim's derriere, his face would assume a puzzled expression that quickly changed to urgency. Fame grew with each spectacular result.

University
Ruperta Carola is the name of Heidelberg University and the home of the "Student Prince." *Gaudeamus igitur* (lets have fun) goes the student song. I intended to do just that. Heidelberg was my first residence away from home and the beginning of a whole new life. It began at a lads-only residence located in Schriesheim, a village outside Heidelberg beneath vineyards and a ruined chateau, the *Strahlenburg*." Disrespectful locals nicknamed our residence the "bulls' cloister." It was a place of male bonding. We drank local wine and sang, listened to Beethoven, Schubert and Wagner, seven or eight crammed into a small bed-sitter, finally free from adult supervision. We cooked blistering-hot curries in the communal kitchen with spices provided by a student from Malaysia. J, the owner of the residence was a man of faith and a natural target of juvenile rebellion. Incongruously he also operated a distillery next door that produced schnapps labeled "*Hochspannung*" (high voltage). It guaranteed a monumental headache the morning after. A few of us swore off hard liquor for life after the experience. We enjoyed provoking J by quoting Nietzsche's "God is dead." His heated defense of the faith became

proverbial as "J's proof of the Lord's existence: "The OEG (tram) can't operate without a *Fuehrer* (leader). Therefor, neither can the world."

J, our *Fuehrer* issued strict rules of conduct, naturally to little effect. Pranks abounded and the strangest hobbies. One chemistry student reproduced *Berger* charges, a combustible mix used in WWII to fog in tank positions. It was launched to the annoyance of hapless farmers plowing fields. Another student issued outrageous decrees in Gothic script. A third memorized train timetables instead of the laws of physics. We partook in street demonstrations wherever one could be found in support of a progressive cause. Having been hit by water cannon became a badge of honor. Two of our mates turned conservative and joined a fencing fraternity. After their first duel they proudly displayed small gashes on the lower left side of their faces, proof of having passed this mandatory rite of passage.

The difference between now and then in the life of university students is striking. Nowadays they learn far more medicine. We learned more about living. Attendance checks did not exist for us. You could stay home, read, travel or go to any lecture you liked, no matter what the subject. I went to lectures on constitutional law and architecture. Anatomy was boring by comparison. Conviviality mattered hugely. This became obvious after I moved into a one-bedroom rental in downtown Heidelberg, miles from the bulls' cloister and all alone. My room was in the old part of town near Heidelberg Castle and pubs. It looked romantic but the reality wasn't. There was nobody around to talk to or cook with and no *Stammtisch*. Cellphones and social media were decades away and dropping in for a visit rarely worked.

After one semester I moved back into the bull's cloister.

The hard reality of medical school began with lectures on anatomy, physiology, physics and chemistry. We shared the chemistry and physics lectures with real physicists and chemists. Lecture halls were far too small for everyone. Queuing was unknown and only the fit and motivated managed to crowd in. I wasn't one of them. Instead I got all the information I needed from friends with notes, a vital connection for those who liked to sleep in. The Institute of Anatomy was forbidding in its own way. An inscription over its classicist portal announced *"Hic Gaudet Mors Succurrere Vitae."* (Here it pleases death to assist life.) No students from other faculties dropped in. It provided formaldehyde-preserved corpses for dissection, one for every six to eight students. The corpses looked like mummies, not life-like like the ones I was to encounter later in pathology. My set of scalpels and tweezers quickly acquired a rancid smell, useful for clearing a table at the *Mensa* (student cafeteria) from squeamish art and law students. I spent an entire week dissecting a hand and learned many Latin names, but not why this mattered. Physiology was less smelly. It taught bodily self-regulation like the feedback loop between the pancreas and the pituitary gland and explained how endocrine disorders develop. All in all, there was an enormous amount of knowledge to absorb before the first set of exams. They culled our cohort by half. This was unsurprising. Getting into medical school had required only a high school diploma. Grades didn't matter. And the courses were free of charge. Seemingly senseless cramming caused students with limited frustration tolerance to drop out early. Tough exams did the rest.

Passing basic science opened the door to the clinical part of medical school, the part that would turn us into doctors. Direct contact with live patients was still limited. I felt restless and decamped to Munich for a change of scenery. Then a budgetary inconvenience developed that required my immediate attention. Instead of asking my parents for more money I got a job at a loo paper factory in Shipping and Receiving. It paid enough to address my budget deficit and broadened my cultural horizons. The factory made soft rolls in white, pink and blue. We started loading them onto trucks at the ungodly hour of eight in the morning. I had to make sure that the correct colors went to the correct village and memorized their postal codes. Around ten o'clock the entire crew went to the pub across the road for a liter or two of brew. Lunchtime brought a second break and more beer. We quit around five, memory being a bit hazy about afternoons. Evenings were a dead loss. I was too tired to go out and my head too fuzzy to read. The initial excitement of being a real workingman quickly faded. Financial health restored, Shipping and Receiving looked like a rut and Heidelberg looked better by the day.

Then came the time to choose a topic for a doctorate, the German *"Dr. med." It* was optional; but my parents had it and so would I. Pathology seemed the very embodiment of scientific medicine, objective and detached from the hustle and bustle of clinical care. My role model was Wilhelm Doerr, Chair in Pathology. He referred me to a satellite institute in Karlsruhe, less than an hour's drive away. The institute's architecture looked like an old North American bank building. It was set amongst trees. Columns fronted its grand entrance hall. 12-foot ceilings, tall windows and neo-baroque ornaments made for an equally imposing interior. Its wood-paneled library was a temple of knowledge. The sweet smell of dead bodies permeated everything. This was the time and place to confront my fear of dead bodies.

The morgue was in the basement, hidden from prying eyes. It housed an enormous stainless steel refrigerator that held some 20 gurneys on rollers. They held the corpses and functioned like drawers in a cupboard. The corpses waited there for their appointment with the pathologist, some still clad in street clothing. The adjacent autopsy room was the size of a small lecture hall. It housed four steel slabs equipped with running water and drains. No sounds from the outside world penetrated there and everything was kept meticulously clean. This was the stage for the ghoulish business of wielding knife and saw on the dead.

Read on at your own risk.

Cutting into human flesh evokes ancient reflexes, even when the corpses don't sit up suddenly. Their only response is passive movement. Seeing a corpse reduced within an hour from being recognizably human to a faceless specimen is a lesson in mortality. We explored every nook and cranny of the corpse to make sure no previously unrecognized abnormality was undetected. The first cut went from the base of the neck down to the pubes. The skin was separated from the rib cage and the abdominal walls retracted. Internal organs were laid bare for inspection. Most were removed onto trays for more detailed examination. Next, a lateral cut split the skin around the dorsal base of the skull, forwards over the ears and downward again towards the chin. This allowed the face to be folded down over itself and freed access to the skull. A circular saw opened it with a screeching noise. The brain was removed and examined. Abnormalities were conferenced with treating physicians and the cause of death declared. Rarely have I seen surgeons look more demure. Afterwards an orderly sewed the corpse back together, cuts hidden skillfully by sutures placed inside skin folds. The corpse looked dignified once again for presentation to grieving relatives.

Relatives had to give their permission for an autopsy unless it was court-ordered. Two court-ordered autopsies proceeded in spite of passionate objections. During the first, relatives camped out on the doorstep of the Institute. During the second, the local rag ran a headline that demanded to know "Who Owns Mother's Heart." A third took place in a funeral chapel in a nearby town. It had been ordered just in time before the actual funeral. The deceased had cut his son out of his will and the son was contesting it, claiming that his old man had been demented when he wrote it. The scene could have been from a horror movie set in ecclesiastic surroundings. We lifted the old man's corpse out of its casket where he had been laid out in his Sunday best, moved him onto a stretcher, cut open his skull and removed his brain, then bagged the lot and left before the mourners arrived for the funeral. The prof was scathing afterwards in his report: There was no macroscopic or microscopic evidence of dementia. And the deceased had written his will "during a lucid moment."

I survived at the institute by sheer grit. Nausea and faintness abated slowly. Nightmares and a sense of despair persisted for months. I lost weight and developed an aversion to meat and to butcher shops that displayed their wares on trays similar to the ones we used for the display of human organs. Eventually I learned to view autopsies from a purely "clinical" perspective, a vital skill in a line of work where most news is bad. Clinical detachment also has a downside. Too much of it translates into an overly detached bedside manner, and that's not what distressed people need. It can also lead to a lack of caution. Close contact with dead bodies is risky. If an infection can kill a patient, it can also kill the pathologist. Precautions at the institute were basic. We used gloves, rubber aprons and rubber boots but no facemasks or goggles. One orderly and one of the pathologists already suffered from tuberculosis when I started. I did not wear a facemask when removing the lungs from two victims of TB. I held them both up by the trachea (windpipe) and filled them with formaldehyde to solidify their tissue. Once solidified, lungs can be sliced thinly and tubercular cavities demonstrated. Both lungs were holed like Swiss cheese, indicative of a severe case. Filling them displaced air and made TB germs airborne, a warning I received only after the fact. Which is how I acquired my very own tuberculosis.

During a visit back home my dad noticed pallor, weight loss and confirmed night sweats. He put me in front of his x-ray machine and diagnosed TB in its initial stage. He prescribed the required medications, breaking the rule of not prescribing for family. His decisive intervention stopped my TB in its tracks, saved my health and my career. I recovered without a trace remaining. It was a close call. TB can be fatal. TB patents were quarantined in the Sixties. Quarantine would have interrupted my studies or scuttled them. I still had to live differently after my recovery, eat regularly to prevent weight loss, go to bed early and rest in the afternoon to prevent exhaustion. I could not party as before. And I had to keep my reasons for this abstinence secret, lest widespread fears of TB might turn me into a pariah. A degree of social isolation was the inevitable result, a lesson on the impact an illness can have over on life style, brilliantly illustrated by Thomas Mann in his novel "The Magic Mountain." I almost took a second hit from TB years later when applying for immigrant status in Canada. Dutifully, I reported my medical history on the requisite forms and received notice that admission might not be granted. Eventually it was granted, but only after medical authorities declared me fully recovered.

In addition to a cure, my medications also provided a lesson in psychopharmacology. One of them turned out to be a precursor of modern antidepressants (the MAO inhibitors). It lifted my mood and turned shyness into extroversion. I felt enterprising and embarked on a stay at the University of Umea in Northern Sweden, this without the requisite Swedish language skills. I am glad I did, or I would have missed out on a truly transformative experience.

I hopped into my VW beetle for the long drive through Denmark and almost the entire length of Sweden, past shimmering lakes, rocky shores and endless forests. In Umea I joined a group of foreign exchange students, one from Communist Poland, one from Yugoslavia and a third from Denmark. Together we enjoyed midnight daylight bright enough to read the paper and a hospitality so generous it was hard to believe. Whatever lectures we attended were held in English. There were smorgasbords, outings to the polar circle, to a mine, factories, a military installation, a stay at a university-owned cottage in Lapland and an overnight sailing trip on the nearby sea. Selma Lagerlof's fable of "Niels Holgersson" added background. (Niels saw Sweden's geographical features and historical sites from the back of a wild goose after a curse had turned him into a dwarf.) My medical studies got short shrift in Umea. There was just too much to see and to do. The visit still had a lasting effect on my career. Umea offered an openness and lack of hierarchical thinking I had not experienced before. I never thanked my hosts properly, much to my regret.

I completed my doctoral dissertation after returning to Heidelberg and devoted its slim volume to my father shortly before his death. It dealt with "bright cells" in the pancreatic ducts of the horse, not exactly a household topic. The cells were thought to be insulin-producers. This had kindled hopes of a new treatment for diabetes. Examining them under a fluoroscope was painstaking work. Photographs had to be taken during the night with the help of a pathologist experienced in the technology. Exposure times lasted hours and even minor tremors from passing streetcars would disrupt the stillness of the image. My research was later quoted in a textbook on the pancreas, shockingly without attribution. Chairman Doerr intervened and my labors appeared in the (German) Journal of Gastroenterology, an unusual distinction for a medical student. They surfaced again decades later in Google Books.

By then new research had dashed any hopes for a treatment of diabetes with "bright cells." They were producing heparin, not insulin.

Preparations for the medical boards consumed my attention afterwards. Clinical detachment numbed grief. The Medical Board exams took place only six months after my father's death. They were exclusively oral and taken in groups of four. Getting together a smart group was vitally important. The schedule was tight, manageable only by soaking ourselves in caffeine. It squeezed internal medicine, pathology, infectious diseases, pharmacology, neurology and psychiatry into just a few months and produced a pressure cooker atmosphere that caused recurrent nightmares in many graduates. Mine were always the same: Exams are approaching and there is a mountain of mandatory reading, impossible to master in time. Thankfully I passed all subjects with distinction except for one career-changing hiccup, psychiatry.

For the psychiatry exam I interviewed a middle-aged woman who had no complaints, not even about being locked up in a ward with barred windows. She was cheerful, talkative, difficult to interrupt and managed to interest me in a stamp collection she hoped to sell. I should have noticed her elevated mood. Instead her interest in collecting stamps swayed my diagnosis. I returned a verdict of obsessive-compulsive disorder, a special interest of my examiner, Dr. Tellenbach. This failed to please. His face grew stern and I feared the worst. Flunking psychiatry with a "5" would have nixed my entire board exam. Instead of lowering the hammer he extracted a promise: I must include a rotation in psychiatry as part of my internship. Under this condition he would give me a "4", which is a bare pass. I promised and he did. Defending my doctoral thesis a couple of months later was a walk in the park compared to the Boards. I was a doctor now, or so I thought. I knew lots of theory and very little about clinical practice.

Internship

In the Sixties Germany required two years of rotating internships before issuing an unrestricted license to practice general medicine. This was a very good idea. Most graduates had yet to learn how to lay sutures, set bones, perform minor operations, deliver babies and write appropriate prescriptions. Obligatory rotations included internal medicine, surgery, obstetrics and gynecology. I remembered my (unenforceable) promise to do a rotation in psychiatry but was not prepared to work on the locked wards of the university hospital. I tried the Max Planck Institute for Psychiatric Research but was turned down in spite of top grades in all specialties except psychiatry. My interviewer recommended "foreign experience." I parked this for later use and decamped to Munich once again, at the time the cultural capital of Germany. Munich is close to the Alps, hiking, skiing, beautiful scenery and the place to be.

My first rotation was in pediatrics in Starnberg, a small town just south of Munich. Rotations in surgery, obstetrics and gynecology and internal medicine followed afterwards in downtown Munich. In pediatrics I worked on an isolation ward for kids with infectious diseases, later with newborns and asthmatics. Some asthmatics recovered quickly after admission and relapsed just as quickly after discharge, raising questions about home conditions. Some parents needed more medical attention than their kids. The newborns often came in as emergencies and in a state of dehydration. In such a case a tiny butterfly needle would be inserted into a vein in the baby's scalp, a fiddly business in the middle of the night but vital, as dehydration can kill a baby.

The next rotation in a private surgery clinic was even better for hands-on practice but lacked supervision. I laid my very first suture there to a girl's forehead while on night call and was overjoyed when no scarring developed during the following weeks. After assisting with a few abdominal surgeries and with the help of an experienced OR nurse I removed an appendix. I anesthetized and intubated (insert airways) and ventilated patients for major surgery, monitored vital signs and learned to cope with sudden drops in blood pressure. Applying plaster casts became routine with only one hiccup, when I was blamed for a poorly healing fracture I had not set. My relationship with nurses and junior staff was friendly. With the chief surgeon and clinic owner it was distant.

A private clinic for obstetrics and gynecology came next. It offered even less supervision. At one point the chief gynecologist and owner was away on holiday and the sole resident physician took ill. I was left to deliver a stillborn on my own, fortunately with the assistance of the father who happened to be a physician. He was calmer than I felt. I also ran the outpatient clinic as no arrangements for coverage had been made. I made sure I did no harm, prescribed colorful vitamins and accelerated return visits. After a weeklong night call came on top of daytime duties I quit an arrangement that would be unacceptable nowadays and completed the remaining gynecology requirement at the university hospital without pay.

There I attended dying women on a cancer ward. They were mostly silent, despondent and sedated by generous doses of morphine. Next came a cardiology ward, also at the university hospital. There some twelve patients waited in one large room in varying stages of cardiac failure for a decisive intervention that never came.

I came away from internship relieved for having stayed the course but doubtful about my future. There had to be something more positive somewhere.

Luck helped with the next step. I had studied from American textbooks for my Boards. With their help and no particular goal in mind I took yet another exam at Ramstein Air Force base near

Frankfurt, the ECFMG. It qualifies foreign graduates to work in US medical facilities.

Once on the base I was herded to a barren-looking classroom with some twenty other candidates. We sat down at rows of school desks and received sheets of multiple-choice questions. These we completed in total silence while suspicious Military Police marched up and down, making damned sure those foreigners didn't cheat. Next I was asked to take a psychological test, the MMPI. My checkmarks must have looked acceptably non-psychotic. I passed the whole thing and qualified for training at an accredited American hospital.

A US military base in Lyon offered the best of all worlds. Located in Southern France, it combined American training with French ambience and the company of locals I had met through my dad. Alas, politics intervened. France quit NATO and the Lyon base closed. In for a penny, in for a pound. I wasn't backing off now and looked for a job across the pond.

Sweden had been great. The US was Sweden on steroids. A brief enquiry yielded multiple job offers, a surgery residency in Hawaii, a neuropathology residency in Chicago, an internship in New Jersey and two psychiatry residencies, one in New York, the other in Florida. All but one were university positions. Which one should I choose, knowing next to nothing about the US? Going back into pathology felt risky. Surgery in Hawaii looked glamorous but was too far from home. The University of Florida was located in a small town and likely friendly. It promised a sub-tropical experience. I made a beeline for it. I listened to "Luncheon In Munchen" on the American Forces Radio in preparation and took an English course. I flunked the course but never mind. One year in Florida would release me from my pledge of a rotation in psychiatry with the added benefit of fluency in English and American training. Opportunities would be plentiful, or so I thought. I hopped on a flight to the Big Apple in October of 1968 with plans to travel south to Florida from there.

New York introduced me to "Hair" the musical, to skyscrapers, a startling degree of social directness and the importance of just going for it. A PANAM stewardess of local acquaintance (sorry, no romance) coached me in the essentials. One thing led to another and eventually to an ad in the New York Times. An elderly New Yorker needed his car transferred to Miami. What better way to go south than to drive his wheels there while taking in the sights? Off I went to a large parking garage in Manhattan to retrieve his car. It was an enormous Cadillac, automatic, air-conditioned and with power brakes that could catapult a novice through the windshield. It started on first try and off I went without hitting anything. That was the good news. Manhattan had absolutely no road signs pointing towards "Gainesville, Florida." After half a day of aimless driving I discovered the value of road maps but not how far it was to my destination. I took the scenic costal route instead of the interstate and took two weeks to get there. I shed woolen layer after layer while heading south and developed a deepening appreciation for air-conditioning.

Arrival in Gainesville confirmed that this was indeed a small town. (It is no more.) I drove into it from one end, went down Main Street, took of few turns and found myself back in the countryside, still looking for the university. I had wanted something completely different and I got it. To the European eye Florida is vast. Cities with wide palm-fringed avenues, long empty coastal roads, flyblown swamps with alligators lurking in the weeds, Spanish moss, solitude and settlers' grit left deep impressions. I spoke enough English to make basic conversation but not enough to make friends. It was tough in the beginning. And then something happened. The place grew on me, the sunsets over the Gulf of Mexico, vast empty beaches, white sand, rustic bars, fried catfish and oysters, whiskey sours, rocking chairs on wooden porches and good ole' boys' Southern humor. Gospel singing to a beat-up piano and rhythmic stomping by the faithful made a small white church rock on its stilts. It was unforgettable.

One experience was straight out of the movies. I was driving my Chevy convertible along the coastal road near Cedar Key, then a fishing village where houses sat on stilts in the waters of the Golf. The sun was setting. A lean man in jeans was relaxing on a porch, his Stetson pushed back to the back of his head. His boots rested up on the bannister and he was having a smoke, the very image of cool. I parked at a respectful distance and put up my boots as well in the back of the convertible. It was so quiet, "you could hear a chicken sneeze" as Woody Guthrie put it in a song. And then, far away, I heard the wail of a police siren. It drew nearer. The man didn't move. A cruiser came to a screeching halt in front of the little house. Two cops jumped out, grabbed their man and dumped him into the back of the cruiser. Doors slammed. The cruiser started up, kicking up gravel. The wail of the siren faded slowly in the distance, silence renewed.

The image seems emblematic in hindsight. There was beauty in it, a hint of ease, adventure and glamor with trouble lurking just beneath the surface. The late Sixties were a time of growing affluence, of Woodstock, an intensifying Vietnam War and protests spreading nation-wide. Florida changed and it changed me while acquainting me with American psychiatry.

2. Which End Is Up?

My first assignment in Gainesville was on a psychiatric ward at the Veterans' Administration Hospital. Mandatory vetting required review of a lengthy list of (probably) communist associations I had never heard of and certainly hadn't joined. I swore that this was true, got my nametag and was introduced to the staff on psychiatric inpatients. Any new job requires adjustment. This one was huge. I was unfamiliar with US drug names and that made prescribing difficult. I had never dealt with veterans before and knew little about the military. My English was too limited for subtleties, let alone Southern subtleties. But nurses, fellow residents and my supervisor helped a lot. I got an introduction to redneck humor and compensatory help with "proper" pronunciation from an English lady. My first supervisor was Henry Lyons, a prof and Air Force veteran who guided my first stumbles with wry wit. He was tall and lanky, sported a regulation crew cut and liked to park his boots on his desk. He wasn't all medicine either, took me fishing in the Gulf of Mexico where we caught grouper, snapper, trout and catfish. And he had a few warnings. "Kuch," he cautioned, "when you find a black snake (a moccasin), don't pick it up." He was exactly what I needed.

One of the nurses was mortally afraid of such snakes. She also liked fishing in a weedy lake. And, being a plucky lady, she carried a six-shooter when venturing there, just in case. Which is how she acquired her reputation as a fast draw. She was drifting peacefully under Cyprus trees when a snake dropped suddenly into her dingy. Startled, she emptied her gun in its direction. Its caliber was large and it holed her boat to the point of sinking.

Most veterans on our ward had recently returned from Vietnam, then a far less benign environment. Our ward was unlocked and they could have walked out any time, another novelty to me. Only one had been admitted against his will. He was a manic-depressive, his latest episode one of many recurrences. His mania (uncontrollably elated mood) had almost subsided by the time I was tasked with his care. The two of us got along like a house on fire, all too well as I was to find out. He was forever cheerful as hypomanics usually are, and I was instinctively opposed to anything authoritarian. Instead I relied on reasoning when he requested a weekend pass. He promised to be good and I issued it without second thought. Equally without second thought, he bought three brand-new convertibles. I was the only one surprised. Fortunately the car dealer nixed the sale and no harm was done.

Most other veterans were admitted for stress-related conditions. They had feared for their life and had seen comrades die. Some had walked "point" in the Vietnamese jungle in conditions of poor visibility and a multitude of perils. "Toe Popper" mines could explode on the trail anytime. Enemies might attack from the front or rear, from behind bushes and out of camouflaged tunnels. In villages foes looked like friends and friends like foes. One warning sign of an ambush was the metallic click from an AK47 being cocked. Ignoring it could mean coming second in a firefight. It was shoot first or hit the deck. One veteran suffered from a particularly intense startle reaction to metallic clicks. This amused his comrades and annoyed him greatly. His hyper-vigilance made perfect sense under Vietnamese conditions. It made no sense at all back home in a country that was at peace. Anxious vets couldn't unwind, slept poorly, had nightmares and became irritable as a consequence. Alcohol and drugs brought solace first and more problems later. Some were withdrawn and kept to themselves. During an outing to a beach near St. Augustine they sat there by themselves, silent and with a 100-mile stare. Detachment was their defense against thoughts of death and destruction.

An even more disturbing aspect of warfare became clear to me years later, when a veteran produced a collection of clandestine photos. They showed half-naked enemy corpses in degrading positions. The enemy hadn't been any kinder to some of his buddies. Psychological warfare like this is nothing new. Mongol warriors practiced it by placing severed heads on stakes to scare the enemy. "Shock and awe" intended to demoralize the enemy at the beginning of the Iraq War. IEDs and roadside bombs returned the favor. The message is always the same, no matter whose side you are on: You are in grave danger and there's no safe place for you to go. Stoicism and emotional detachment may shield against some of this but at a cost. Once back home, ongoing wartime detachment impedes re-engagement. Family, friends and coworkers feel distanced, even rejected by a veteran who is edgy and preoccupied. The veteran in turn feel will abandoned. Nobody understands. Worse than that, Vietnam veterans who had risked their lives for their country felt betrayed. Public hostility to the Vietnam War and "warmongers" included them who had no choice in the matter except for desertion.

I tried to engage my veteran patients through discussion. They were always polite, addressed me with "sir" as if I were an officer and stayed formal. The language barrier and my limited understanding of their concerns didn't help. I was a greenhorn and a stranger. I knew little about psychotherapy beyond the need for empathy. And I had yet to decide which school of psychiatric thought I would follow.

There were four major theories to choose from, organic psychiatry, psychoanalysis, psychobiology and behaviorism. Organic psychiatry (genetics and brain injury) was not as much of a focus as it is now. Psychoanalysis and psychobiology seemed to explain a lot but had little to say about the treatment of acutely troubled people. And behaviorism was still in its infancy. As a wag once put it, two Adolphs were to blame for the "lamentable state of American psychiatry." The first one was Adolf Hitler who chased the psychoanalysts across the Atlantic. The second Adolf was the Swiss psychiatrist Adolf Meyer. He imported the notion that anxiety and depression were "reactions" to stress (while excluding other possibilities). The diagnostic classification of the day reflected this assumption. Behaviorism offered impressive experiments like Pavlov's dogs (that learned to salivate in response to the sound of a bell) and Skinner's boxes where rats searched for rewards. But it lacked clinical application.

Soldiers used their own remedies during the wars. German WWII troops used the amphetamine Pervetine to combat fear and fatigue. British pilots used similar agents during the Battle of Britain. In Vietnam American soldiers self-medicated with cannabis to get away from it all. I had less at my disposal. Tranquilization and emotional support were my only remedies. It was like fighting a dragon with a toothpick. Could a more sophisticated kind of psychotherapy work? I was ready to experiment.

Gainesville's training program offered a variety of psychotherapeutic orientations. They included psychoanalysis, Rogerian psychotherapy, behaviorism and Gestalt therapy. Psychoanalysis required years of training analysis and took far too long with its clients. Carl Rogers believed in "unconditional positive regard" as the main agent of change. An animal experiment seemed to support it, if ever so slightly: Deprived and "depressed" young monkeys were introduced to "monkey psychiatrists." These "psychiatrists" clung to the deprived monkeys who then got better. Clinging to a client and uncritically supporting everything she might do looked unappealing. I wanted a more specific technique. Our behaviorist George Barnard was more practical with his hard-nosed observations. He taught us what to look for. And Gestalt groups were engaging. So why not try one of these or even both? And there was more to try, if only to satisfy curiosity.

Wilhelm Reich's "Orgon therapy" was considered very fringe even in the wild and wonderful Sixties. But I liked Ollendorf, Reich's son-in-law who was in Gainesville as a visiting prof from Germany. He was blunt and really funny, recommending "re-odorization" to meticulously deodorized staff. According to Reich's theory, Orgon therapy improves orgasm and relieves neuroses. That's a win-win. Excessive muscle tension was the Orgon version of Freudian resistance to change. It needed breaking to open a client up for progress. I decided to have a go, no matter how odd this seemed. Obviously I was too "resistant" and Ollendorf "broke" me for an hour or so by stretching my shoulders and hip joints to their physiological limit. I got away sore but unconvinced.

Vincent O'Connell was a Gestalt psychologist who ran an encounter group for psychiatric residents. It offered a forum for conflict resolution and personal growth. We met weekly for an hour-and-a-half, sat in a circle and the brave ones "let it all hang out." Whatever happened in the group stayed with the group, just like Vegas. *Gestalt* is a German term meaning figure or shape. As a therapy it demonstrated blind spots in one's perception of oneself and others, thereby bringing their *gestalt* into view. To accomplish this we had to be "authentic," to say exactly what we saw and felt and then "take responsibility for it"(instead of blaming mom and thereby blurring the *gestalt*). Volunteers could turn up the heat on themselves, take a seat in the "hot chair" inside our circle and have a go at self-exploration. I had been brought up to never "make a spectacle of myself" but also wanted to learn. Out came homesickness and a longing for "the green, green grass of home," not exactly a revelation. I didn't want to go maudlin' and stayed clinical, as if describing a third-party case. Eventually Vincent asked me to talk face to face to one group member and tell him how I felt "right here and now." This was closer to the bone and led to a few disclosures and a good weep. Afterwards I felt strangely elated, clearer and a little less alone. A series of sessions improved my comfort with close scrutiny and receiving unfiltered news about myself. I also became a better interviewer, got a feel for discomfiture, evasion and touchy issues that bothered my peers.

More groups followed, this time with me as a facilitator. Stetson College invited John Renick, Rock Cheshire and myself to run groups on their campus south of Gainesville. We soon realized that some students were too fragile and anxious for an intensive encounter group. The psychological literature reported breakdowns. Fortunately none of our students suffered one, but it seemed to be a good idea to investigate further. John Renick and myself designed a study. Molly Harrower, a psychologist and senior faculty member offered testing for a pre- and post assessment. For this Molly used the Rorschach test, a projective method that uses inkblots and is rarely used nowadays. She had developed a quantitative method of scoring it to test US Air Force pilots. Our results from the student group suggested a degree of positive change. None got worse. Improvement was non-specific but good enough for a pilot study and publication. A control group and measurement of changes in students' daily lives would have been needed to come to any solid conclusions. Our groups were part of a general trend. A highly mobile society had made relationships more transient and generated a need to make friends quickly. Encounter groups provided a training ground for this. They lowered barriers to intimacy and encouraged directness. Spontaneity was considered more authentic than careful deliberation and sober second thought. That was seen as too "controlling." Nowadays we ask if all this spontaneity made society more confrontational. The groups also provided a counter-measure to emotion-based opinions. They included role-play and, most importantly, role-reversal. For the latter we changed places with our partner in the group and role-played him while he role-played us. We then coached our partner until he represented our point of view adequately and he did the same with us.

Just imagine Republicans doing this with Democrats; it would be quite a party game.

After six months at the Veterans Administration I moved to a psychiatric ward at Shands Teaching Hospital. It held civilians from all walks of life, some "psychosomatic" ("physically ill" without a physical basis). My duties included care of a woman with debilitating headaches who had not met diagnostic criteria for migraine. She kept to herself, spent most of her time in bed and was moody. The "therapeutic milieu" of the ward was intended to relieve her (presumed) stress. Unfortunately, discussions with doctors, support from staff and fellow patients, good food, music and art therapy didn't help. Gestalt therapy was a non-starter with her. After all, she already had a headache. I was stumped and wanted better answers, beginning with a more medical approach.

I undertook a rotation in neurology back at Veterans Administration. It taught me how to conduct a proper physical examination, to perform a spinal tap and other invasive techniques. It covered, dementia, paralysis and pain. I was impressed by the research going at the VA on sleep encephalography and alcoholism. Kurt Freund's drunken mice were fascinating. They were "just like your old friends." They subdivided into three groups when offered a nozzle that released an alcoholic drink. Some took a brief nip and declined drink after that. Some really liked it but only in moderation. And some stayed glued to the nozzle and went completely blotto. Chronic headache remained a puzzle.

Earlier on Shands' psychiatric ward a young woman had presented yet another challenge. She refused to leave home unless her parents accompanied her. Our "working diagnosis" was schizophrenia. I ran the gamut of looking for stress and parental "ambivalence" according to Bateson's theory of schizophrenia. His now obsolete theory postulated a "double bind" by mixed messaging from mother to child. It said "yes" verbally and "no" non-verbally. Double messaging was thought to confuse the child to the point of psychosis. I scrutinized the patient's mother and found nothing of the kind. I was stumped again.

Fortunately the behaviorist George Barnard offered a different take. He sidestepped any diagnosing and asked what told me specifically that something was wrong. That was obvious enough: She never went out alone. "Then," he said, "why don't you go out with her and see what happens?" I ignored dire warnings from a psychoanalytic supervisor and did exactly that. My patient and I went for a walk. She did not become psychotic or "act out." We went out for more walks and increased our range. She got better, I don't recall to what extent. She was probably agoraphobic and agoraphobia improves with desensitization.

The experience became my guiding light: Stick with what you see, describe it and connect the dots. In Western movies their hands tell you if they'll draw. Words are mere ornaments there. Behaviorism works the same. It sticks with observable events where two different sets of eyes can agree on what they are seeing. Nothing else is added until all opportunities for further observation are exhausted. Description comes first. Opinion comes last. That cuts down on speculation that cannot be tried and tested.

To recap: Our young lady wouldn't go out alone. Anyone could see that. Accompanying her outdoors proved that she could. She just wouldn't go alone, but why? She looked nervous at the prospect. Why was she nervous? What could go wrong if she went out alone? Could she identify a threat? No, she couldn't. It did have a location, the places she wouldn't visit on her own. I took her there, first onto the hospital grounds, then into groups of people and open squares. How close did I have to stay to maintain her sense of security? I could check her pulse to see if her heart was racing, indicting nervousness. I could step away from her until she asked me to come closer. And I just like anybody else could observe changes in her range of travelling alone and by how much it improved as we progressed. Just about everything was verifiable within this behaviorist approach.

3. Drugs and Medical Wards

"Don't Bogart the joint my friend, pass it over to me" went a Sixties song. It was cool then to smoke up, particularly on campus. Timothy Leary came to lecture. Sitting cross-legged under a palm tree he encouraged us to "smoke up, expand your mind and grow." At a rock concert with Janis Joplin cannabis smoke hung thickly over the crowd. Bulky cops wandered through it to catch offenders but caught none. "Roaches" vanished quickly under a flap of sod before a "pig" could get near. Very respectable people also did it and gathered around water pipes that made them giggle while risking jail. It was a confusing time. President Nixon would soon declare his War on Drugs and fill his jails while Canada's Ian Cameron (reportedly) experimented with LSD at the behest the CIA. To residents on emergency call one thing was clear. Cannabis was keeping us busy. Freak-outs were common amongst students who had forgotten "not to inhale." They rushed to the emergency room, hoping to be "talked down." This took more time than we residents had. A solid dose of Valium (Diazepam) was faster but disliked by those who wanted a "soft" landing. Eventually users became more sophisticated and the number of emergencies dwindled. Perhaps some also realized what risks they were taking by fooling with their neurotransmitters.
Much has happened since. The decriminalization of cannabis is slowly repeating the stepwise lifting of Prohibition. Canada and several US States decriminalized its medical use as a first step. Then, as before with alcohol, prescribing practices loosened. Eventually, as with alcohol, government discovered the benefits of taxing the stuff. Eventually, the Canadian Government decriminalized it for recreational purposes and now supplies it in licensed stores, again just like alcohol but with a health

warning. In the US, legislation varies from State to State while also moving in this direction.

A medical ward was the place for my first encounter with alcoholism, not the rowdy variety but the quietly hidden kind. I was working on the consultation service when a medical ward at the VA urgently requested an opinion. My patient was bedridden in a private room. He was thin, pale, restless, confused and exuded a fruity smell. He denied all substance use. His medical workup had been negative and I couldn't pinpoint any reason for his mental impairment. I scheduled a second visit with my supervisor Mike Kehoe, an Irishman wise in the ways of the world. Mike had a quick word, sniffed the air and opened the bottom door of the night table. Out tumbled many empty bottles of aftershave. The source of the fruity smell and confusion was revealed, also the role that evasiveness plays in such cases. After a few years' practice I never asked about alcohol use directly. Instead I asked about drinking prowess and how many drinks someone could hold. This yielded more accurate results.

Few medical and surgical patients welcomed visits by consulting psychiatrists. Many feared that such a visit might discredit their symptoms as "psychosomatic" (meaning imaginary) and consented only reluctantly. Being sick is always "psychosomatic" when you think about it. It's distressing to experience medical symptoms, the discomforts of hospitalization, separation from family and friends, financial strain and not quite knowing how this will end. Resulting distress can be severe enough to aggravate an illness and delay recovery. Consequently psychiatric consultants have to cover three diverse areas, mental health, physical health and socioeconomic background to fully understand what is going on. Particular diplomacy was required in the Sixties for a sexual history. You didn't ask directly, especially not in the old South. With a lady it was barely proper to ask: "Does your husband still bother you, mam?" With men the approach could be more direct. However circumspection had gone AWOL when I offered advice to a man of the cloth in true Gestalt fashion. Performance anxiety had caused his impotence.

He worried about failing and rejection. In my considered opinion he needed to focus instead on his desire and on the anatomical feature where he felt his desire most. He had to "be his penis," a suggestion I uttered with Germanic gutturals. A puzzled look developed on his face, then an expression of patience and forgiveness. Our therapeutic relationship did not blossom.

On night call at the VA the "Officer of the Day" had to cover all specialties, medical, surgical, neurological and psychiatric. Fortunately psychiatric emergencies outnumbered all others and no life-threatening illnesses came my way. Senior physicians were unenthusiastic about being woken in the middle of the night but helpful in crises. A law student filled in as nighttime administrator and a shoulder to cry on. His hobby was tracking veteran "snowbirds" that frequented northern VA hospitals during the summer and migrated to southern hospitals in fall in search for a bed. He received his alerts from further north and in turn alerted colleagues further south to impending arrivals. He also sent out an alert when an enraged snowbird choked me in the middle of the night. The snowbird wanted a bed and now. He didn't care for hours of talk with a Kraut, having seen quite enough of them overseas. He came at me with claw-like hands and grabbed my throat. Fortunately he was unarmed and I was young and fit. The two of us got into a bit of a dance and made a lot of noise until help arrived. He was cleared medically and spent the night on a hard cot in jail, not what he had been looking for.

At the VA hospital emergency room I had to see all comers. On night call at Shands I only had to see psychiatric emergencies. This was far more relaxed but could still be lively. One of my first cases was a young lady with full-blown mania. She had directed traffic in her birthday suit at a downtown intersection. Cars were coming to a screeching halt until police rushed in. She was clad only in a blanket that the nurses had draped over her to prevent another display of charms. I admitted her against her will and in a hurry. A Justice of the Peace had to be phoned to ok this. A time-honored procedure followed: "What's up doc?" the Justice asked. I explained. "That's ok then, doc" he replied and hung up.

At Shands, residents weren't just there to learn. They were also asked to teach. I volunteered to enlighten student nurses, expecting an informal occasion like a small round table or focus group. Instead I found myself on a brightly lit stage in front of a large hall filled with chatty students. An American flag stood to one side and the whole thing looked frightfully official. I wasn't used to public speaking and sweated buckets. My heart was racing and I had difficulty breathing as I held my notes with trembling hands. But I survived. One nursing student even told me that I was "cute" as I hurried to the exit. This (lecture) experience led me to experiment with medications. I was prescribing them. So why not try them myself? Diazepam slowed my palpitations when I lectured again and eased the feeling of breathlessness. Out of curiosity I also tried Amitriptyline (Elavil), the antidepressant of choice at the time. It flattened me and made me feel "spacey." Chlorpromazine, the anti-psychotic of choice for emergencies was very sedating. Trifluoperazine (Stelazine) had an emotionally steadying effect but made swallowing difficult. – I have listened closely to complaints about side effects ever since.

4. Esalen and the Student Health Service

The Student Health Service was located right on campus in a small office building. It offered free one-on-one psychotherapy with psychiatric residents. Two senior staff provided supervision. Our clients were vocal, informed and a joy to talk with. I could be as busy or un-busy as I wanted to be. During lunch breaks I played tennis, frequented the well-stocked university bookstore and read piles of psychology books. The cat had fallen into the cream. The books offered a smorgasbord of philosophies and techniques.

There was Colby's associative interviewing, the kind that's used with insight-oriented psychotherapy. The interviewer homes in on the most significant aspect of a client's statement and follows it up with his next question, question after question. Eventually this gets to the heart of the matter, be it fear, loss or love affair. It worked well with thoughtful students, less well with students who were anxious and needed guidance. Glassner's "reality therapy" could be more appropriate there. It confronts clients with the hard facts and challenges them to solve their problems themselves. Erich Fromm's "Sane Society" is more sociology than psychiatry and takes the opposite view. Social problems make people ill. A sane society would be less competitive, more supportive and de-conflicted. Karen Horney explored social conflicts inherent in women's social role, the requirement for them to be competitive on one hand and "nice" on the other. Her therapy seemed written for the Southern lady of the times who was always "really nice," sometimes through gritted teeth. It meshed well with assertiveness training, a technique designed to help shy people. Eric Berne's "Games People Play" explores interpersonal transactions and what they imply. Transactions can be on the same level (respectfully "adult to adult"). They can be domineering and dismissive (belittling parent to uninformed child) or the reverse, pleading and talking up (submissive child to parent). Recognizing and realigning transactions would de-conflict relationships. Fritz Perls' "Gestalt Therapy Verbatim" was different again and the blueprint for our residents' encounter group. It focused on why you worried NOW, why you CHOSE to worry instead of doing something about it and instructed you to TAKE RESPONSIBILITY for your choice, to "own it" as we call this nowadays. It was more behaviorist than explanatory, offered a psychotherapeutic technique worth trying and I wanted more. Fritz Perls had founded Esalen, a Gestalt institute at the California coast south of San Francisco. It offered courses and John Renick suggested that we apply. We were accepted and the University funded our excursion with jaw-dropping generosity. Sadly, Fritz Perls died just before we got there. But the courses continued and we departed full of anticipation.

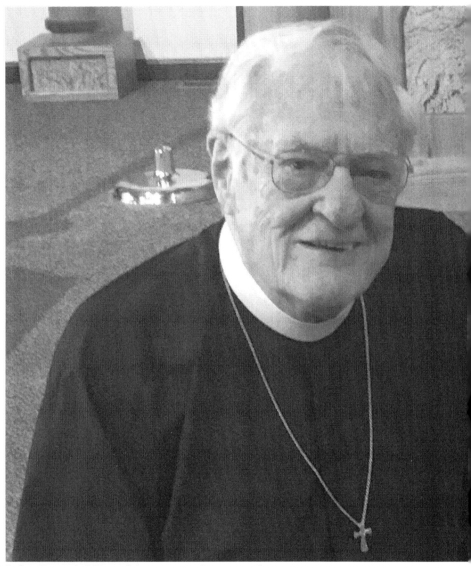

John Renick MD in his current incarnation

San Francisco had what the movies promised, breath-taking views across the Bay, colorful neighborhoods and many cool people. Everybody seemed to hang out and hang loose. We hadn't been there for a day before a stranger invited us to a party with lots of drop-ins who told you their life story.

California wines, the sounds of Santana's "Black Magic Woman" and Mungo Jerry's "Summertime" got us fully into the groove. Having recovered from the party, John and I hired a big sedan and hit the road a la Jacques Kerouac of "On The Road" fame. We headed south on California's Highway One without a plan, tasted local wine, slept in the sedan and listened to the surf. The sight of a breast-feeding woman greeted us at the gate to Esalen. Esalen sits near the edge of steep cliffs. A cool wind blew up wispy mists when we arrived and large waves crashed into shore below. Seals and sea lions were hanging out down there and we were soon hanging out above, feeling as one with nature. Hot tubs provided conviviality and cold showers were there for those in need. Sharing your feelings came naturally in a setting where lessons on nude massage taught deep relaxation. The lessons were paradoxically repressive. A little voice in the back of my head told me that visible signs of male interest in the female participants were definitely out of bounds, particularly from professionals. I pinched myself whenever the need arose (behaviorists call this "thought stopping") and studied the female bodies on display exclusively for signs of illness. We flew back to Florida after two weeks of encounter groups, feeling extremely laid back. My new self got rid of his tie, the single sartorial feature that had identified me as hospital staff. Bell-bottom jeans and a T-shirt replaced it. Nobody seemed to mind except for my British supervisor Mike who considered this "improper."

At the Health Service, students worried about the draft and Vietnam. I wasn't but should have been with my immigrants' visa. Some students hoped for an exemption by being labeled "gay," back then a psychiatric diagnosis. I sympathized and called a congressman on behalf of one particularly distraught draftee. He lent a sympathetic ear but had no further comment. Some time later the American Psychiatric Association removed homosexuality from its list of Mental Disorders (DSM) and with it this particular escape hatch from the draft. Change was in the air in many other ways. Signs marking "colored entrances" were fading over rural facilities. Our first black medical student

entered Shands Teaching Hospital under police protection.
Friends moved away, John to California and my teacher Vincent
to Toronto. My favorite cinema closed and I lost access to
European art films. I felt foot-loose and still a bit homesick for
Europe. Toronto had felt more "European" when I visited
Vincent there, so why not try it for a year, even if this meant
leaving paradise? After all, I could always come back.
Vivian Rakoff at "The Clarke" (later re-named CAMH)
interviewed me when I applied. I turned up in full California
mode, in bell-bottom jeans and one day late but precisely at the
appointed hour. He grumbled, but I was accepted. Maybe
Toronto was short of applicants. Then two going-away presents
made parting from Gainesville even harder, the "Anclote Award
for an outstanding residency" and the publication of a second
paper on psychotherapy. They made me realize that I was
leaving a great university with excellent career prospects. I was
leaving behind more than that. I was leaving those long, lonely
roads to the Gulf and the Atlantic, the Island Hotel of Cedar Key
where Bessie, innkeeper, retired sociologist and Mayor of town
mixed her Island Sour Whiskeys and fried her crab cakes. I was
leaving a wonderfully laid-back way of life, my teachers and a
good many friends. But off I went, feeling homesick for Florida
almost as soon as I arrived in Toronto. I was sorely tempted to
return after passing my American specialty exams. And I did
many times, but only as a tourist.

5. Toronto Here I Come

Montreal had been my first choice amongst Canadian
universities. It had the Allan Memorial Institute, cafes, wine bars
and old-world charm. Unfortunately La Belle Province didn't
want me unless I served another medical internship and passed
another set of Medical Board exams. To make matters worse,
both had to be in French and I was far from fluent. Ontario was
more welcoming. Ontario Boards were in English. My German
internship and American residency training were recognized
there. I had to serve one more year of residency to qualify for

Canadian specialist certification. That was no problem. It would help me adapt and give me time to plan more long-term. I briefly considered returning to Germany, but North-American residency training wasn't recognized there. Job openings existed but not at universities and I was not in the mood for more serfdom. The only doubt I felt was about the frigid Canadian climate. My US immigrant visa had expired when I emigrated. To keep my options open I went to the US Consulate to apply. The Consul was flabbergasted. "What are you doing up here?" he asked, then helped me out of this particular bog with a multiple re-entry visa. With this up my sleeve I settled down for one more year of residency. Toronto had museums, an opera house, expat communities from all over the world, a great university, a multitude of beautiful lakes, the Canadian Shield and the Algonquin Park further North. I could do a lot worse.

The powers that be assigned me to St. Michael's Hospital in downtown Toronto, starting January 1972. St. Mike's had a timeworn charm with neo-gothic architecture, nuns in starched habits and a cafeteria that smelled like a granny flat. It was like the *Diak* in my old hometown. Nearby was the Eaton Center, a very urbane mall with a domed glass ceiling that became invaluable later for the treatment of agoraphobics. A Greek hole-in-the-wall restaurant invited me into its kitchen where I selected a flavorful lunch from pots bubbling on the stove. In an Italian dining hall waiters wore Roman togas. The Underground Railroad offered Southern food. A German *Gasthaus* combined faux Tudor with kraut piled high besides schnitzels, ham hocks and sausages. Weight gain seemed inevitable.

The department at St. Michael's was less eclectic than Gainesville but tolerably so. Insight-oriented psychotherapy was king. Other approaches were tolerated but not taught. Gestalt raised eyebrows. Residents practiced "formulations," a somewhat ritualistic description of the intra-psychic mess of desires and conflicts that we supposedly harbor. We studied the diagnostic manual of the American Psychiatric Association (DSM) and diagnosed according to its criteria. My early efforts attracted little critical acclaim. I failed to see the point of classifying anything beyond the treatment it required. Only distinctions between psychosis, depression and neurosis made sense. Psychotics got antipsychotics and support. Neurotics got anxiolytics, antidepressants and psychotherapy. The dismissively labeled "worried well" received analytically oriented psychotherapy. Typically they were high-functioning people with enough time for thoughtful self-examination. Senior staff saw most of them. The urban poor and people with somatic (bodily) complaints fell to the residents.

Walk-in clinics with multidisciplinary staffing were a novel and very promising approach to the care of the urban poor. In New York Arnold P. Goldstein's "Structured Learning Therapy: A Psychotherapy For The Poor" had introduced such a clinic. John Salvendy started one at St. Mike's. "The Wednesday Clinic" was located across the street from St. Mike's in a disused chapel and combined psychiatric, occupational and social services.

The limited scope of psychiatry stood in stark contrast to the work of the "real doctors" who had lab tests and x-rays, surgery and antibiotics. We had nothing of the kind. Thankfully some cracks showed through their seeming omnipotence. Diabetics did not follow a prescribed diet. Cardiac patients refused rehabilitative exercises and acute care patients left hospital against medical advice. Lack of cooperation and inexplicable symptoms baffled even the most brilliant neurologists. My first assignment was on the psychiatric consultation service, the place where psychiatry and medicine meet and sometimes clash. Fortunately I had related experience from Gainesville. Donna Stuart, then our chief resident, later Chair of Women's' Health and recipient of the Order of Canada showed me the ropes. She became a good friend and improved my diplomatic skills in a territory where I, the consultant, knew less medicine than the physicians who sought my assistance.

My first challenge then as before was to gain patients' trust and demonstrate that I was there for a second look. "Four eyes see more than two" was the mantra. Consulting was a detective's job that looked anew at a problem from every angle. Why was a drug "not working?" Was it not taken as prescribed? Did it cause side effects the patient did not dare complain about? Why might a headache, bowel symptoms or palpitations occur under some circumstances and not in others?

On one memorable occasion the hospital environment turned out to be the culprit. A boy had suffered severe burns on a large part of his body. After a week's confinement to a bed in the intensive care unit he developed worsening confusion and restlessness. I sat down besides the heavily bandaged lad, gave my name and explained what I was trying to do. He was wide-eyed and terrified, didn't know where he was, where his parents were or what time it was. Instinctively I re-oriented him. I explained what nurses and doctors were doing and why. After half an hour of this he calmed down and began to talk more coherently. I felt like Moses on the mountain. His problem was sensory deprivation combined with sleep loss in a noisy ICU that had no windows and no other indicators of day or night. A multitude of monitors were beeping. Staff was rushing back and forth amongst patients who were in various stages of agony. Subsequently staff provided the lad with a watch and took care to maintain his orientation. Modern ICUs are better at keeping people oriented. They provide daylight, a quieter environment and semi-private beds whenever possible.

Night call is the bane of every big city resident. We endured it on a rotating basis, sleeping fitfully in a Spartan duty room until the phone jolted us awake. You could watch yourself getting conditioned by the calls. After a few jolts I only dozed in anticipation of the next call until dawn greeted my bleary eyes. Even angels get testy when sleep-deprived. One night a novice operator patched through yet another call. A voice declared, "I can't sleep." "Now I can't sleep either" was my unsympathetic reply. St. Mikes is in a part of town that harbors social problems galore. Threats of self-harm and suicide were common. Drunks abused staff but couldn't be turned away until a thorough examination established that this was safe. This was the psychiatric resident's job. She had to talk to people who didn't want to talk to her but to "a real doctor." She had to calm troubled waters, determine the odds for something going wrong and provide the rationale for a safe discharge. Beds were scarce and admissions appropriate mostly for depressives and schizophrenics in crisis. When admission was unavoidable and beds were full, residents spent a lot of time in the middle of the night, bargaining with other residents at other hospitals for a bed (in my jaundiced view really the job of hospital administrators). And on the following morning their exhausted and frustrated selves returned to "normal duties."

My second rotation of the year was on "inpatients." This was familiar territory. Medication, supportive group therapy, occupational and social services and the "therapeutic environment" was all we could offer. Crises had to be defused and everybody be kept happy, not an easy job with people who are unhappy by definition. On one occasion the police brought in an arrest with a bad leg. He seemed barely able to walk, then suddenly lost his limp when nobody was looking. He was an Oscar-deserving actor who made his escape to a waiting get-away car. The police detective was unhappy with our guardianship and threatened charges. It fell to me to point out that an open psychiatric ward is not designed for holding hardened criminals.

Adjusting to the climate and a big city, cramming for Ontario Medical Boards and Canadian specialty exams dominated my first year in Toronto. The great outdoors had to wait. The specialty exam would anoint me as a fellow of the Royal College and get me some respect. It wouldn't solve a larger problem that kept nagging. Upon completion I would have six years of medical school, two years of rotating internship and four years of residency under my belt. And in spite of all this, a rude German pun about medial specialties still had a ring of truth to it: "Surgeons do a lot but know nothing; neurologists know a lot but do nothing; and psychiatrists know nothing and do nothing." The answer to my problem was hiding somewhere in plain sight. It took a while to find it.

6. On Staff at St. Mike's

Moving up the totem pole to a staff position meant more money and more respect. Passing the general medical as well as the Canadian specialty Boards added two more feathers to my cap. Passage of the American specialty Boards in New York added a third. The university added a fourth by appointing me lecturer. Now that I had the headgear, how would I fit in? Would I publish or perish? I was no longer on a salary and had to make a living through fees. Bluntly put, that meant going into business. Kurt Weil was (almost) right: *Erst kommt das Fressen, dann die Moral* (The grub first, morality later). It wasn't quite this harsh; but economies do shape the delivery of healthcare and departmental politics.

Chiefs of university staff hold sway over assignments, office space, salaries and academic promotions. By implication, they hold say over staff time and where it is spent.

A psychoanalyst occupied this hallowed ground at St. Mike's. An inner circle shared his priorities and supported his decisions. Psychiatry Associates, fondly known as "Psychotic Associates," ran the business end of the department. Associates included all staff psychiatrists regardless of seniority. It distributed all funds earned through direct patient care and through supervision of resident-provided care according to a formula. Psychiatrists who provided more services made more money, up to a pre-set limit. Lecturing medical students was not a clinical service and wasn't remunerated. By taking time away from billable work it translated into a financial penalty. With perfect logic, junior staff gave most of the lectures.

Associates provided a forum to discuss ongoing business and decisions made higher up the food chain. We were like the United Nations. Two Aussies, one Hungarian-Austrian, one Yugoslav, one Canuck who had been raised in Trinidad, two Brits and one German held sometimes frank and open discussions. Battle lines formed between junior and senior staff, contained by Roberts's Rules of Order. The seniors held most of the cards but not always. On one occasion the chief required funds for a special project. Just like Congress, Psychotic Associates had the power to defund it, but only by stealth and by the creative use of Robert's Rules. Unnamed conspirators placed a bonus payment to all members on top of the meetings agenda, juniors and seniors alike. It was approved unanimously. Such motions always were. Passage mopped up all excess funds, including those for the project championed by the chief. The conspirators looked suitably surprised when the agenda finally came to the chief's project towards the end of the meeting. There was no money left for it.

Psychotic Associates never reached the resourcefulness of parliamentary committees. But it provided a lovely training ground.

Money wasn't the only ticklish issue. Patient care was another. Psychiatrists who chose insight-oriented psychotherapy as a mainstay of their practice prefer a client that's introspective, educated and vocal. But there's downside to this. Too many insight-oriented psychotherapists may end up chasing too few "suitables" while the "unsuitables" lack a place to go. The latter include people with psychoses, severe anxiety, depression and inexplicable "psychosomatic" symptoms. Fortunately several staff psychiatrists broke through the impasse. Josip Divic's brief health questionnaire shifted the focus away from insight-oriented interviewing (where the patient receives little direction from the interviewer) towards a more medically oriented approach to symptoms. Donna Stewart's work in Womens' Health had similar priorities, as did John Salvendy's walk-in Wednesday Clinic reduced disruption of care by no-shows, a common problem with the urban poor and facilitated their adherence to treatment. It also took care of the financial penalty that no-shows would otherwise inflict on doctors in a fee-for-service system.

I also opted for a predominantly medical approach and opened a headache clinic within the mental health clinic. Unfortunately this wasn't a departmental priority. The headache clinic was closed twice "for lack of space." Finding a confrere in Richard Swinson for my interest in behavior therapy helped a lot. We ended up collaborating for decades in three different hospitals, first at St. Mike's, then at Toronto General (TGH, later part of UHN) and eventually at CAMH (originally the Clarke Institute). We met with other behaviorists from the greater Toronto area who supported each other in an environment that did not support behaviorism and poked fun at Freudian orthodoxy.

Eventually Richard and I moved our practices to TGH Toronto General Hospital). There Richard's administrative skills and an eclectic chief of staff (Alastair Monroe) allowed us to start officially Canada's first university-based Anxiety Disorders Clinic. It had existed unofficially before at St. Mikes. At TGH it grew into a focal point for research on anxiety disorders, nationally and internationally.
Later on Richard became Chair of Psychiatry at McMaster University.

7. Investigating a Headache

Remember the headache lady from Shands? Her pain was so severe that she retreated to bed in a darkened room. This is not unusual. Millions have that problem. The cause was often unknown when I came across it first and medication was of little help. Later at St. Mike's, more headache patients were referred to my office, frustrated, discouraged and questioning the idea that a psychiatrist could be of any help. A few were willing to try something, anything, to find a way forward. And so was I. The problem was that there was nothing obviously abnormal to see (apart from complaints of pain). Therefor there was no clear path towards a remedy. But I kept looking and looking until I bumped into a big surprise.
Two theories of headache seemed worth a closer look at the time. One was a theory about tension headache. The "monkey in the rain forest" illustrates it best: It hunches its shoulders against foul weather. Supposedly we humans do the same when we habitually tighten our neck muscles in adversity. When this

hunching becomes chronic, so the theory goes, neck pain and tension headache develop. In migraine the mechanism was thought to be different. There vascular constriction was considered the culprit and cold hands were a sign of it. If this vasoconstriction (constriction of blood vessels) could be prevented, so this theory went, an episode of migraine might also be preventable. (Note the multitude of "ifs.") I needed monitors to display these processes, one for muscle tone and one for peripheral temperature. A variety of monitors were available. Particularly interesting was one crime investigators used, the so-called "lie detector" that tracks change in respiration, heart rate and sweating in response to probing questions. Sudden peaks in these variables reveal what questions get a suspect stressed. Similar monitors might tell me what was going on with my patients. But the idea of using this in headache was untried and unlikely to attract the funds necessary to buy the pricey medical equivalent of a "lie detector." I had to find a poor man's solution. Help came from a laboratory in Montreal that sold "biofeedback" equipment as the technique was called in the Seventies. It was basic. But it monitored muscle tone, peripheral skin temperature and sweating. Besides monitoring it also fed back to the subject how she was doing. It was exactly what I had been looking for. It would reveal changes in muscle tension and peripheral temperature in real-time. Feedback of these variables might train volunteers to control them and maybe, just maybe, their headaches as well. The hospital research committee was justly skeptical. After some back-and forth it funded the purchase of a temperature and a muscle-tension monitor (EMG) for a pilot study. I added a monitor for sweating (galvanic skin response or GSR) from my personal funds. Now I was off to the races.

We use real-time feedback every day when we shave or apply makeup. Only the monitor is a mirror, not a sensor. Try without and you'll realize how much control real-time feedback provides. For temperature feedback I attached a temperature sensor to an index finger and connected it to a monitor. The monitor buzzed with a pitch that increased as temperature increased. That closed the feedback loop. My volunteer could literally hear her finger warm up and see it happen on a visual display. I was my first guinea pig and a successful one, raising my temperature by some seven degrees after an hour or two of trying. So did most volunteers. Monitoring muscle tone was equally straightforward. I attached EMG electrodes to the dorsal neck muscles and the forehead while my subject relaxed in an easy chair. The pitch of the feedback sound from the monitor increased whenever muscle tone increased. My volunteers learned to relax, some a bit too well. On occasion you could hear a gentle snore emanating from the lab. Clearly, people could be trained to control these two "autonomous" functions.

How about controlling headaches? Quite a few migraines and tension headaches did improve. But here's the rub. Headaches wax and wane regardless of treatment. Such a natural up and down is typical for most chronic illnesses. It also generates a second pattern: People seek help when they get worse. And when they get better they believe that treatment helped, even when it didn't. Their improvement occurred as part of the same up-and-down pattern that had made them worse initially. This "regression towards the mean" (automatic return to an average over time) creates a tendency towards erroneous beliefs in ineffective therapies. I had not designed my trial to exclude this possibility. That would have required a baseline (average symptom levels before treatment) for comparison against treatment effects. I would have required a control group as well, one that was blind (unknowing) if it received a placebo (fake) treatment or the real deal. Bottom line: I hadn't corrected for bias. By itself, this wasn't major flaw. Many pilot studies are done this way. But without convincing results a retrial that would meet these stringent requirements could not be justified.

Failure is grist for the mill. Learn and move on. Galvanic skin response (GSR) monitoring was my third window for a closer look at puzzling symptoms. It became useful by chance. A patient agreed to try the GSR sensor during an exploratory interview. When connected, the monitor emitted a ticking sound that sped up and got louder whenever her sweating increased. We talked about neutral subjects at first and the feedback sound didn't change much. Then we moved on to family matters and the slow tick grew to a high-pitched scream. I changed the subject and the scream subsided. I changed back to family matters and it returned. Something discomfiting was going on at home, something she hadn't disclosed. Little was known at the time about the physiology of anxiety and the nature of fears and phobias. All of a sudden this little black box offered a means to demonstrate an anxiety she had tried to ignore. It also demonstrated to her that her anxiety had physical consequences (and by implication that "psychosomatic" did not mean "imaginary"). And then I got really lucky: I tried the GSR with accident survivors.

Fast forward to the Eighties. I was riding the subway on my way home when a man nudged my ribs and pointed meaningfully at a woman napping on a seat. She was his spouse, he said and I had treated her nine years earlier with success. Eager as always to learn about a success I conducted a follow-up interview on the spot, results separately confirmed by Jean Martin, our nurse at the mental health clinic and guardian of the coffee maker. Jean had assisted me nine years ago when I treated the woman. The two kept in touch subsequently, thereby creating the kind of follow-up most therapists can only dream of. In the seventies her complaint had been head- and neck pain after a car accident. Biofeedback did not help, but she believed that her anxiety in traffic aggravated her pain. Logically, I suggested that we get into a car to check this out. The idea terrified her. But she was prepared to do it under sedation and in the company of her (then) boyfriend. I gave her a strong dose of an anxiolytic. Jean and I then half-carried her to my car and drove her through traffic for some two hours. I took a few Polaroid snaps for documentation. On follow-up she had little recollection; but the Polaroid shots convinced her that she could do it again. We repeated the procedure with a lower dose of the anxiolytic, then several times more under declining doses until she travelled medication-free. Long-term success was nothing short of dramatic. She became able to travel without restriction. She also believed that her pain was better.

This was breaking new ground. Over the following decades I replicated the procedure with other victims of traffic accidents. Most managed without sedation. Their fears improved. Pain usually didn't. Years later I collated my observations with similar observations Richard Swinson had made, then published them. Publication of a treatment manual followed and a screening test for "accident phobia" and PTSD (The Accident Fear Questionnaire).

One of my colleagues, Bill McCormick, published a description of declining dose desensitization. Subsequent research has shown that exposure therapy (direct confrontation with feared situations) is more effective without sedation. Unfortunately, many phobics feel too terrified to try it unless an anxiolytic is offered. Declining dose desensitization is a compromise that gets people into exposure therapy, not an adjunct treatment. One piece of advice to those tempted to try this on a friend: Don't do it without the help of an experienced physician or psychologist. Exposure therapy is demanding. Its success depends entirely on the willingness of its subject to confront fear repeatedly and for extended periods of time, each time without interruption until fear has abated; or your phobic will get worse. Exposure should also never be attempted by surprise and never without informed consent. And it is only as good as the behavioral assessment that preceded it, as I will show below. In other words, not everything is a nail when you hold a hammer.

Some of my clients remained fearful no matter how much time we spent on the road. Then it was back to the drawing board to find answers to the obvious question: Why did they fail to desensitize? More precisely, what exactly did they fear in the first place? One example was a classical back-seat driver that shouted warnings to his driver. He desensitized only after agreeing to ride blindfolded. It was essential that he surrender control. A statistical analysis of some sixty cases revealed this as a common pattern: Most nervous accident survivors fear riding as passengers more than driving a car themselves.

Some driving fears had nothing to do with accident phobia. A fear of driving across bridges and over an exposed hill turned out to be agoraphobic in nature. Another client (who had been in multiple accidents) happily surrendered control, contrary to the usual pattern. She feared driving when she was at the wheel herself. Logically, I asked her to do the driving when we went for a test drive. She then had me on the edge of my seat during a series of near misses. This wasn't something I could treat. Instead I referred her to a course in defensive driving that covered safe lane changes, proper separation from other cars and avoiding a "box" of surrounding vehicles that would place her at their mercy.

On another puzzling occasion I served as vehicle inspector. A "floating feeling" was making this driver feel unsafe. It turned out to be realistic. His vehicle had wobbly front wheels. Attempts at desensitization would have been worse than useless.

8. The Frights

Fast forward again, this time beyond the year two thousand. I had treated flight-phobias for years and always wondered what it would be like to experience a fear of flying first hand. And then my wishes came true. I the therapist got the frights myself. That's embarrassing, but also a unique opportunity to describe the experience from the inside and from the outside, from the point of view of clinical experience.

How did this happen to me? The ancient Greeks blamed panic on the god Pan. I blame mine on "preparedness," on my long-standing unease about enclosed places and two prior anxiety episodes on planes.

I got the frights briefly in the Seventies on an unventilated plane. Four of us were at Santiago airport shortly after Pinochet came to power. The airport was chaotic. Passengers were trying to get a flight to "anywhere, just out of here." After an anxious wait and with a bit of luck we finally boarded our flight. The plane was nearly empty and didn't take off as scheduled. Instead it sat on the tarmac in the boiling sun with doors closed. There was no air conditioning and the inside became stifling hot. I began to feel short of breath and panicky, then switched into clinical mode and watched the goings-on with detachment. Eventually the plane took off and I relaxed. The rest of the flight was uneventful and I forgot all about it afterwards. More years passed without further mishap. Then I had another episode. One early morning I was flying home from San Francisco after celebrating with family the night before. We parted early in the morning and I rushed to the airport, loaded with caffeine. Once on the plane I got suddenly anxious while it was still taxiing. Anxiety passed after takeoff and I forgot all about it again. Nothing further happened until just before retirement. That's when the frights really struck. I was flying home from London Heathrow early one morning, again after a goodbye celebration the night before. Again, caffeine had helped me through the rush hour. While the plane was taxiing I felt a sickly twinge of fear in the pit of my stomach. The plane took off and my fear faded. Then it returned in force and I couldn't dismiss it. I had the same thought my clients used to describe: "What if I can't stop this? How much longer 'til arrival?" Fear continued to grow. I was like being sucked into an undertow of terror. I felt faint, breathless and had palpitations. I tried to disrupt this and went to the washroom to splash my face with cold water. That worked briefly. Then the next wave hit and I felt pulled under once more. Fortunately training and experience kicked in. I was going to use what I knew from treating clients.

I was feeling closed in and short of air. I countered by inhaling and exhaling from the depth of my stomach, slowly, as if asleep. A blast of fresh air from the ventilation system helped some more. I resolved to stay put indefinitely, relaxed neck and shoulders and tried to get into a book. This worked, but the frights returned whenever concentration slackened. I knew they wouldn't kill me, but it sure felt like it. And then it dawned on me that focusing on how I personally felt was part of the problem. A reality check was readily available: Everybody else on the plane looked perfectly relaxed. What I felt wasn't imposed by my surroundings. Nothing had reached inside me to cause this existential dread. It was of my own making, from associating confinement to a small place with flying and associating both with a threat of asphyxiation. I had to break this association by reasoning, by counteracting it with relaxed breathing and by treating anxiety as if it was part of the furniture.

I got through the flight all right, then realized it had brought on the "fear of fear" that Claire Weekes described so well: Nobody in his right mind would want a recurrence of this ghastly feeling. But there's no way to guarantee that this won't happen unless one stays home. That lack of a guarantee creates a paradox. The more I worried about it, the harder I tried to prevent a recurrence, the more I would be attentive to the slightest twinge of fear. And that could trigger the frights all over again.

A story made the rounds in the early days of behavior therapy. Someone with a severe case of the frights was getting depressed and suicidal. Most of his episodes occurred in open squares when he was alone. They felt like dying. He decided to put an end to it all and went to the worst possible place he could think of, a lonely hilltop. Once there he waited to die. And nothing happened. He had defeated the paradox that a fear of fear creates. He had stopped running. His technique is now known as "flooding with paradoxical intention," basically a way of saying "bring it on." Years later a woman called a CBC radio talk show with exactly the same idea. She also suffered from a bad case of the frights. She also was convinced that she and everyone like her had to deal with the fear of fear by accepting a possible death to get over it once and for all. To most people this seems a bit harsh. Might it be possible to tackle the frights indirectly, through cognitive strategies?

Lets begin with a dose of reassurance. Might you lose control completely and "run screaming down the isle?" This is one of those thoughts that intense fear can generate. The answer is "probably not" (which is the best you'll ever get in medicine): I don't know of a single case where this has happened. I have never seen it described in the literature. And by chance, I watched three fellow travellers who were in the throes of the frights. They sweated buckets and two were hyperventilating.

None "lost it." They just sat there and endured. Loss of self-control seems to require an added element of surprise. Richard Swinson and myself searched our combined records for such cases and found only a hand-full amongst hundreds of phobics. None had a fear of flying. One jumped out of a moving car because he discovered a wasp. Another ran into a wall and suffered broken ribs when a dog surprised him. A third jumped from a boat to get away from a wasp, although he couldn't swim. These cases had one thing in common, the element of surprise. Flights are different. They are planned ventures and surprises are exceedingly rare.

What exactly do flight phobics fear? That varies. I don't like enclosed places and confinement. That's claustrophobia. Agoraphobics fear flying because they don't like being far from home and from their "safe" place. In the Seventies Air Canada allowed an agoraphobic client and myself onto the flight deck of a parked Boeing 747 and explained safety procedures. It didn't help. Safety was not her worry. Being far from home was. But our visit to the cockpit might have helped a disaster-phobic, someone who worries about crashes when engine sounds change and aircraft wings wiggle.

Can anything else contribute to the frights? I believe so without being able to prove it. In one study on panic disorder close to one-quarter of the volunteers improved before enrolment to such a degree that continuation with the trial became pointless. What had happened? Maybe they felt better after having the whole business of the frights explained. They had also abstained from alcohol and caffeine for two weeks. Maybe they felt better because of that. Alcohol withdrawal can cause jitteriness even after moderate use. Too much caffeine can do this too. Phobics are already on a hair-trigger before a flight. Conceivably both substances may lower their resistance even further. A few days' abstinence certainly works for me. My flight preparations also include an unhurried departure and keeping my "emotional temperature" down.

I have also carried an anxiolytic on board. An adequate dose can terminate the frights. Just carrying it reduces the "fear of fear"

and I never needed to take it. Beyond that it's flying, flying and more flying until you forget all about the frights and get into a book or movie after the doors close.
I guess I am just like my patients.

Anxiety disorder isn't limited to a fear of flying. It comes in many shapes and guises and affects some eighteen percent of the North American population annually. It is the most common psychiatric disorder in the general population (NIMH). And yet it doesn't always get recognized. Anxious people like to keep their condition private. Most just clench their teeth and get on with it. Panic disorder is a particularly severe form of anxiety disorder. In the USA and Europe its one-year prevalence is around 1.7% (NIMH). I like to call panic disorder "the frights" because it implies less in the way of biological disease and more in the way of cognition and behavior. Both play a major role in it, as demonstrated by the role behavior therapy and cognitive strategies play when managing it.
People get the frights in all sorts of places, in crowds, on social occasions, with public speaking and when faced with small animals like mice, cats, snakes and bats. The frights represent a survival instinct that's gone wild like a bolting horse. It pops up in the wrong places and for the wrong reasons. Back in the Stone Age it may have made sense. It was dangerous then to be separated from the clan, to be surrounded by strangers, go into strange places all-alone and confront unfamiliar animals. People with PTSD also experience the frights but are more in tune with modern reality. They get their frights "triggered" by reminders of a severely frightening experience.

Below an additional note on agoraphobia, the most common variety of severe anxiety disorder.
In 1871 the German psychiatrist Westphal described how agoraphobia starts: Three young men experienced sudden inexplicable terror, then developed fears of empty streets and the "*agora*" (the Greek term for meeting place). As so often in science, Westphal's paper was received without full recognition of its importance. It took a century before it was rediscovered

and considered as a diagnosis in cases of seemingly inexplicable symptoms. (Remember my young lady at Shands?) Agoraphobia can be crippling. Some agoraphobics become housebound. Some need a trusted companion to feel secure. Some depend on such a companion to such a degree that they never spend any time alone.

Mild agoraphobia may not be this obvious. It can remain undiagnosed until something happens that demands a major adjustment. This can be a change at work that demands more travel and more time away from home. It can be a medical disorder that is anxiety-sensitive like irritable bowel, asthma and heart disease. And then a vicious cycle can develop as one aggravates the other.

The subway was one of the most feared places amongst my Toronto clientele. My companionship made it relatively "safe." For purposes of treatment I would first sit right next to a client, then further and further away, eventually on the next train near the end of treatment.

Therapist-assisted exposure can work for entire groups and in different scenarios. The Eaton Center in downtown Toronto offered a whole menu of sites that agoraphobics fear, crowds, heights, elevators and narrow passageways, all perfect for exposure therapy. Group treatment offered economy of time and the added benefit of mutual encouragement between clients. Independent practice without the reassuring presence of a therapist or companion was mandatory before "graduation." Without it the need for support cannot be broken. Success means being able to do whatever matters to you without undue distress. This could be travel all over Toronto, all over the Province or all the way overseas. To name one shining example: One agoraphobic had been unable to travel alone beyond the downtown core of Toronto. He wanted to work abroad. And he did. Some years after we had parted a small parcel from Down-Under arrived to prove it. It contained an ancient fossilized fish inside a stone. It's still on my desk. What made the difference between such a smashing success and minimal progress? Only a small percentage of clients accept exposure therapy as full-fledged as this man did. It requires great fighting spirit and never forgetting why one is in the fight. A therapist can encourage and push. Only a vision of a better future provides the pull that assures that a client does go all the way.

Exposure therapy and cognitive behavioral therapy (CBT) were our bread and butter and the Anxiety Disorders Clinic at Toronto General Hospital, one of the first if not the first in Canada, founded in 1981.

9. What Will People Think?

My gran worried a lot about "what people might think." Her worry sums up this chapter in one single sentence. "You must always leave a good impression" was her other way of putting it.

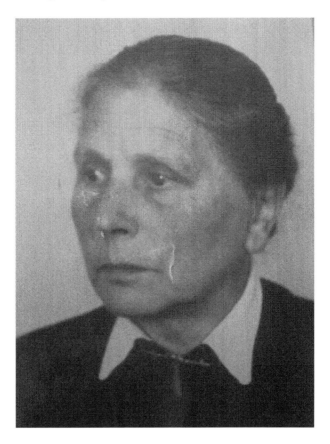

My gran Anna, looking concerned

The popular Britcom "Keeping Up Appearances" takes gran's concern one step further. The lead, Mrs. Bucket, doesn't just worry. She wants to change minds. She wants her name pronounced "bouquet," tries for a posh accent and pushes her candlelight dinners on important people who would rather be elsewhere. In keeping with Alfred Adler's theory about the inferiority complex, she over-compensates for feeling inferior by acting posh. An entire industry caters to our desire for social status. We spend billions to look fashionably thin, donate good money to dine with celebrities and hope to get on the news. It's a harmless sport in moderation, counter-productive when overdone. If you talk too much about yourself as Mrs. Bucket does and over-dress, you are only advertising the fact that you don't belong.

Social phobia takes these natural concerns to a much higher level. Mrs. Bucket persists with her efforts because she can. A social phobic can't even try. He gets the frights.
The DSM sums up social phobia as a "fear of negative evaluation." It's normal to worry about a job interview and normal to look anxious. A reasonable interviewer won't mind your trembling hands unless you are looking for a surgery position. Trouble starts with the idea that you absolutely must look right and talk right or disaster will strike. What's required to reach this level of perfection and why the penalty of failure should be so severe is in the mind of the beholder and only there. Someone else wouldn't care. Usually perfection requires a don't. Don't blush, sweat, tremble or stutter, not even one little bit, or else. And here's that same paradox again, just as with fear of flying. The more you worry about your particular horror, the more likely it becomes. Suppose you are on a date and fear blushing. First you blush ever so slightly over some minor embarrassment. Then you fear that your date might notice and blush even more. Looking embarrassed embarrasses you. And then you want to run and hide. A similar mechanism operates

with sweating, trembling and stuttering. The harder you try to look cool, the worse you get. You know this of course and that it makes no sense. But you can't shake off this unwanted preoccupation.

One shaker couldn't write well enough to sign a check in front of a teller. This was before the days of on-line banking. She feared the teller might notice her tremor, suspect fraud and call the police. The more she tried to control her shakes the shakier she got. She had to send a confidante to the bank with a cheque made out to cash. Why shaking should be so utterly unacceptable was unclear to her. It just was. Compare this to the attitude of a friend of mine with Parkinson's disease. She shakes badly because of her disease. She may not be happy about it but, as far as she is concerned, that's just too bad. She even teamed up with a few others who also have Parkinson's. They call themselves "the movers and shakers" and raise money. They are role models. To get over a fear of shaking you need to flaunt it instead of hiding it. It's very hard to do this, but it can be done.

Sweating is similar. I remember an executive who wouldn't wear a light colored suit even on hot summer days. The fabric might stain and show him up as a nervous wreck. At the clinic we sprayed his armpits with water until stains showed. He tried this out and came to realize that nobody cared.

One aspect of social anxiety is practical. It's lack of reliable feedback. My gran worried about what people think. And she couldn't possibly know what they thought. That meant that she was flying blind. She might try to read facial expressions and body language, but there are too many ways to misread these, particularly for someone who is anxious. The only solid feedback is based on behavior, on what people do. Will they talk to you again, call, invite you and make an effort to keep in touch? Or are you the one who makes all the effort? For treatment purposes that means only one thing: Forget about what people might think. That's the space for your worst phantasies. Instead, keep your eye on what they do.

Fears of public speaking are almost universal, with certain aspects to them that are completely normal. You want to please, but there's little feedback. Remember though that your listeners are probably just like you. They won't care about small mistakes and nervousness unless you get outright cringe-worthy. Practice helps. Hiding doesn't. Reputedly, Bernard Shaw cured his fear by stepping on a soapbox at every opportunity. He also had something to say. If you don't, your nervousness is realistic. If you don't rehearse you'll stumble. One of my guiding lights, the Chair on Pathology at the University of Heidelberg was famous for his lectures. They looked ad lib, but he rehearsed them and how. You could sometimes hear him shout his upcoming lecture from the washroom. Nervousness before parties and dates is equally realistic. You expect to be scrutinized. You make contact by making conversation. That's anxiety-provoking if conversation skills are lacking. Conversation is like playing Ping-Pong. Lead off with a question like "been to the film festival?" Comment on the answer, then ask the next question. Be ready with a number of topics. She-Who-Knows-These-Things recommends researching the interests of new acquaintances for suitable topics. Still anxious? Finding rejection hard to handle? Role-play dating with a friend. Reverse roles, see what it's like to be on the receiving end of your efforts and practice until put-downs and haughty silences loose their sting.

A full-fledged social phobia can look like a medical problem on first sight. Some performers get dizzy and fear falling. Some public speakers feel that cannot draw breath. A groom had a more unusual problem. He came to see me before his wedding because he "couldn't swallow." His GI specialist had ruled out physical abnormality. When asked about the when and where, he described how he couldn't swallow whenever he was the focus of attention. The upcoming wedding presented a lifetime challenge. He had to bring a toast to the bride from the head table with everyone looking on. Then he had to down his drink. And of course it should be perfect. Treatment was twofold. First came education: Actual choking is extremely rare in healthy people; feeling like choking is fairly common with the frights.

Next came exposure and practice. We met for small lunches at my office and swallowed together, using a hierarchy of increasingly "difficult" foods. We started with yoghurt, moved up the scale to salads, progressed to hamburgers and finally to stringy beef. He practiced at restaurants and that got him through his wedding.

Treating social phobias often is like coaching. It also requires foresight. In my early days as therapist I obtained the consent of several women to meet at a small restaurant in a private corner. They all feared conversing and eating with strangers. I promised that there would be "no pressure" and lots of mutual support. All agreed, seemingly enthusiastic. I felt confident after earlier successes with individual therapy and booked a table at the restaurant. My chaperone Jean Martin and I arrived there, got to our reserved table, sat down and waited. And no one showed up. Thus ended one of my larger lessons on social anxiety: My clients wouldn't say "no" to my face. They were too under-assertive and I hadn't considered this possibility. None came back for another try.

An old German saying makes a great line for people who fret about appearances: *Und ist der Ruf erst ruiniert, lebt man gaenzlich ungeniert.* (Once your reputation is ruined you won't feel embarrassed ever again.) Unfortunately this doesn't work for performers. Ordinary mortals may have every right to make a hash of it. They can fluff their lines. Performers can't afford to. They may no longer feel embarrasses. But they will be poor. The MP3 player has made life hard for musicians, as Tim Harford observed in his book on " Fifty Inventions That Shaped The Modern Economy." Before the MP3 player's arrival many live gigs were on offer even to mediocre performers. Then all the money went into recordings and now you have to be top drawer to make a buck. As a movie star you live under the microscope. You worry not only about performing. You also have to develop the right kind of public image. When faced with such pressures, how can public personalities cope? And what can treatment accomplish? It's tough. Imaginary exposure (a form of CBT) to worst-case scenarios and rehearsing how not to give a damn helps sometimes. Having developed a "plan B" in case the worst happens can be reassuring. Medication may help some more with a bad case of the frights. "Dutch courage" probably doesn't.

No discussion of social fears would be complete without a mention of the nether regions. Men had the starring role in my practice. The "pee-shy" syndrome" is well known amongst urologists, judging by referrals. It befalls mostly young men who feel mortally embarrassed by the sounds of a healthy stream splashing against the walls of a urinal. It might be overheard and that's embarrassing. One student clammed up completely unless privacy was guaranteed. He dreaded written exams because all visits to the washroom were closely monitored, to ensure that there's no cheating. He avoided caffeine and liquids to help his odds. Still, there was no guarantee he wouldn't have to go and this worried him to distraction, literally. He couldn't concentrate on his tests. His behavioral treatment required joint visits to the washroom after cognitive preparation. To ensure voiding he took a diuretic. Neither one of us liked it but the smelly visits worked.

Below the belt lurks yet another fear that haunts men, the fear of being unable to "perform." It's usually worse with new partners and with demanding ones. Apologies for bluntness, but there's no such thing as being scared stiff under such circumstances. In behavioral terms, "psychogenic" impotence (without underlying illness) results from competitive inhibition: the response to the inhibiting stimulus (the fear of failure to "perform") wins out over the sexually arousing stimulus. Sexual response is not a command performance, no matter how hard you try. It's like the flow of saliva. Either you are keen on what you see and relaxed enough to enjoy it or you aren't. One unfortunate fellow had the worst of it. At a red-light establishment circumstances were unattractive, to say the least. They elicited only faint arousal. And to his partner time was money. The balance between arousal and anxiety was all-wrong and passion failed to bloom.

Similar principles govern sexual response in women. In anorgasmia, emotional and physical discomfort may compete against sexual arousal and win unless her partner is considerate. And a bad experience can create a hangover that lasts months or years. That could be because of pain (dyspareunia), or fear or both, as in sexual violence and rape.

10. Psychological Trauma

From the outside the military looks glamorous and daring. As seen from the inside, it also exposes you to the risk of psychological trauma. The German Army offered me a brief glimpse of this reality when it "invited" me to join the tank corps after graduation from high school. Participation in a maneuver was meant to demonstrate how exiting military service could be. Dutifully, I answered the call, went to the base and climbed into a tank of Korean War vintage. It had a huge cannon, was deafeningly noisy inside and lacked a suspension. We rumbled out of the gate and entered a large field with many humps and bumps. And then the beast broke down as we came over a hill. Command declared us "technically dead." I didn't like it, but didn't lose my boyish interest in war and its machinery. Years late the same interest led me down the narrow entrance of a US diesel submarine, this time only as a tourist. The experience made me wonder how anyone could spend months and years in such narrow confines while charges exploded all around. War may be entertaining, but only if you are not in it. The veterans in Gainesville made this perfectly clear, as did American and Canadian veterans I assessed years later for service-connected injuries in Toronto.

A tail gunner I examined on behalf of the Canadian Army suffered from persistent anxiety ever since the War. When cannon fire from a German fighter cut the intercom of his bomber it severed all communications between him and the surviving members of the crew. Suddenly he was all alone and isolated in his perch while his bomber limped slowly back across the Channel. He knew nothing about the state of the pilot and his chances of making it home. The bomber barely cleared the cliffs and crash-landed in a field near shore. He emerged physically unharmed. Then recurrent nightmares set in and claustrophobia that troubled him for decades.

A commando also suffered lasting psychological injury. He led a platoon in the battle of Monte Cassino in 1944 when his men surrounded a farmhouse occupied by German defenders. The Germans refused to surrender and fought back for days. They killed one of his comrades and then ran low on ammunition. Overwhelming firepower finally killed them. The commando returned home a silent man. He kept reliving the firefight and barely spoke for decades, except for the most essential utterances. He worked, but only alone and in a menial capacity. Surprisingly he spoke to me at length. Even more surprising was his empathy for the German defenders. He broke down in tears as he described their courage and their death and took some time to calm down.

A US veteran became severely anxious after surviving a mortar attack on a large medical facility in Vietnam. Unarmed soldiers scrambled for cover as mortars began to fall in the middle of the night. The perimeter was breached and the base was on the verge of getting overrun. Help seemed far away. Fortunately the attack was repelled, but it was a close call. The veteran felt on a hair trigger afterwards, jumpy and alert for noises in the night. He booby-trapped his Toronto flat against nighttime intruders and wouldn't enter parts of town where Asians lived. This seemed like paranoia, except that my company relieved his fear. His defensive reflexes hadn't transitioned from then to now.

A Canadian Special Forces soldier retired from peacekeeping service sometime after a RPG had dealt his armored car a glancing blow. His life took a downward turn. He became moody, irritable and couldn't sleep. One night he fell asleep on the Toronto subway. He claimed that two TTC employees "kicked him awake." He came to with a start, looked around, saw them standing over him and went berserk. He was good at it. Both suffered injuries in the one and only assault I have ever seen committed by a veteran. He was let off after I submitted a letter in his defense.

The Canadian General Romeo Dallaire served as a peacekeeper through the horror of the Rwandan genocide. His memoir describes in detail its psychological impact and consequences to his health. War was a life-changing experience, to him as to may others. Torture victims risk the same. One impressed me by his impassive attitude. He was a Somali who complained of pain and nothing else. He remained impassive even when he told his story. He had been forced to run behind a jeep with his hands tied to the vehicle to the point of utter exhaustion.

Police offers are also not immune to psychological injury and PTSD. They get bitten by dogs, swarmed by crowds, have guns pointed at them, examine bloodied victims of traffic accidents and murder. Traffic checks and walking the beat can turn dangerous at a moment's notice. I had lunch with one officer who changed his seat to have his back face a wall. Sitting with his back to the entrance "just didn't feel safe." A veteran of a SWAT team suffered from persistent nightmares about a suspect in his gun sights. He had been ordered to pull the trigger in case of armed resistance to protect civilians and other officers. Visibility was poor. He wanted to fulfill his duty but felt uncertain if he was aiming at the right man. Another former SWAT member faced down a suspect that drove a truck at him while he was on foot patrol. He faced a reprimand for drawing his weapon "prematurely." Disciplinary action was withdrawn after his psychological state received due consideration.

Rape also leaves deep emotional scars. Choking is particularly terrifying. The victim can't breathe and can't know if the chokehold will be released in time. Fear of death is the inevitable result. Safe and unsafe situations can be hard to tell apart after a rape, particularly after acquaintance rape. If it happened once it can happen again. How can a rape survivor tell with any certainty who's safe to date and who isn't after an experience like that? Of course it makes sense to avoid anything risqué like alcohol consumption, drinks of unknown provenance, abandoned parking garages and deserted streets. This improves the odds but guarantees nothing. Any stranger on the street and any date could be another wolf in sheep's clothing. Some rape survivors deal with risk by ignoring it altogether, as if challenging it. Some call this a counter-phobic attitude. There's one clue though that shouldn't be ignored. The rapist Paul Bernardo enjoyed extreme domination before strangling his victims. A jealous husband in Newfoundland stabbed his spouse to death while shouting "you are mine." Both wanted total control. Both wanted to "own" their victims. If a date seems controlling, domineering and coercive, beware. You don't want him to "own" you.

Many of the above examples raise important questions. When does extreme fear cause lasting damage? Who is more vulnerable and less likely to recover? I asked myself these questions many times, first when the German Consulate retained me to assess Jewish concentration camp survivors on behalf of German Courts.

11. Nazi Concentration Camps

Nazi concentration camps exemplify the cruelty of racism in its most organized and lethal way. Their construction began in 1933 after Hitler came to power. One of the first was Dachau near Munich, followed by some sixty-seven others. Initially the camps housed political prisoners, gays, gypsies and mentally disabled persons. Then Jews were confined there in ever increasing numbers. In 1942 the SS leader Heydrich chaired a meeting of senior Nazi officials known as the *Wannseekonferenz* in a palais near a lake in Berlin. The palais is now a museum commemorating the planning of the holocaust. Senior Nazi officials put together organizational details for the "final solution" to the "Jewish question" there. The Jews of Europe would be rounded up, confined in camps, forced into hard labor and ultimately "exterminated."

An estimated six million Jews succumbed to the camps, to exhaustion, illness, starvation and poison gas in purpose-built chambers. Eleven million non-Jews also died in the camps (according to the Washington Holocaust Museum). Deportations were conducted under the guise of "re-settlement" to newly conquered territories in the East. Deportees were taken there in locked cattle cars. A substantial number did not survive the journey. All this is widely known and sometimes denied. The film "Schindler's List" reminds us of the horrors of camp Krakow-Plaszow in graphic detail. Auschwitz/Birkenau was apparently worse. Upon arrival there detainees were "selected" for slave labor under the cynical motto of *Arbeit macht frei* (work liberates) or sent directly to their death in the gas chambers. Those who survived the selection were tattooed with an identification number beginning with an "A" (that resembled a triangle) on the volar side of their left forearm. Some underwent potentially deadly medical experiments under the direction of Dr. Mengele, a hardline Nazi doctor. Near the end of the War many detainees died during death marches while driven west as the German army retreated. Small memorials now dot the German countryside to commemorate these marches.

After the War the Allies confronted the German public with the realities of the holocaust and a "collective guilt" that was not easily forgiven. Villagers who lived near former camps were confronted with the evidence. School children (including myself) watched footage from Auschwitz shortly after its liberation. Footage included the gas chambers, barracks with impossibly crowded sleeping quarters, dazed survivors looking skeletal in striped uniforms and corpses piled high. In the early Fifties the *Bundestag* (parliament) passed several laws for restitution (*Wiedergutmachung*). One law restored stolen property to its original owners. Another compensated Jewish survivors for medical and psychological damages sustained in the camps. Arrangements were made for claimants who had moved overseas. Their compensation was determined in part on their hypothetical earning capacity that would have existed, had it not been diminished by racist persecution. Claimants had to document their incarceration and its duration. The German State retained local physicians to provide the required medical assessments. And German courts adjudicated the matter.

In the late Seventies (or early Eighties) a fellow staff member from the Department of Obstetrics and Gynecology at St. Mike's (Charles Luttor) contacted me on behalf of these courts: Would I be willing to provide psychiatric assessments of concentration camp (KZ) survivors to determine their eligibility for restitution according to German Law? The court files were in German and would provide proof of KZ stay and its duration. That would take care of the burden of proof as far as Nazi persecution was concerned. Only the nature of claimants' symptoms, their severity and their impact on work and career development needed to be assessed. Anyone who had been in a camp for one year or more was presumed to suffer from psychological trauma, unless proof of an alternative cause was evident. The German government provided "guidelines" for assessors. I would be function as a "Friend of the Court" and be accredited in Frankfurt, Muenchen and Berlin. I would be paid a modest fee for each case. Court appearances would not be required. Charles Luttor provided such assessments in his specialty. The interviews were "difficult" he said, even for him with his Hungarian heritage. They would be particularly difficult for someone with a German name.

My first applicant arrived at St. Mike's with a paralegal in tow. The paralegal deposited his briefcase on my desk with an audible crash and began to quiz me on my knowledge of the holocaust. I was getting my first experience with an adversarial situation. After hearing him out, answering some of his questions and accepting supporting documentation I relegated him to the waiting room. My claimant then cooperated. I took a long time over the next few days to write up my first report.
Getting quizzed about holocaust denial was perfectly acceptable, especially in a medico-legal context and when ongoing holocaust denials add insult to injury. I was prepared for that. I was familiar with footage from the camps, had spoken with my dad about the holocaust and his chance encounter with an execution squad. At university I had been a member of a German-Jewish friendship group. In Sweden I had met a Jewish exchange student from Poland who described how the holocaust had

surprised her family. Feeling an affinity to German culture and science, they had refused to see the threat. But this was new. It took me a while to realize that I was not just a doctor taking a history. My role as assessor made me a representative of the country that had committed these atrocities.

Assessors have feelings too, just like everybody else. I harbored guilt and shame for "being German." Other nations had also committed atrocities. But the Nazi camps were as bad as could be, and two wrongs don't make a right. It's been alleged that certain cultural traits enabled German atrocities. Was this true and did I harbor these? I had learned as a child to resent the wanton exercise of power. It took me longer to question the indifference and fear that enabled the holocaust. My only defense was the accident of birth. None of us choose our ethnicity and how we are raised, not Jews, not Germans, not anyone else. Conduct deserves scrutiny, ethnicity never. That wasn't all. I also had to guard against my anger at being accused of something I hadn't done, anger that could bias me against a claimant. And I had to guard against the opposite, against favoring claimants out of guilt and pity in the absence of supporting evidence. I needed to develop an assessment protocol that defeated bias and in a hurry. This may sound unfeeling, but the alternative would have been opinion based on emotion instead of fact. Sleepless nights drove home this point. Fortunately recently acquired research skills came to the rescue. I developed a protocol based on psychological tests and a semi-structured interview and followed it consistently. It made assessments more elaborate than required by the Courts but also better. By the end of my appointment I had assessed some seven-hundred survivors over three decades. Their stories changed me and my convictions. If the holocaust happened once, it can happen again. Racism of any stripe, ethnic cleansing, the remnants of Stalin's Gulag, Chinese re-education camps and the Rwandan genocide make this more likely, particularly if we blindly believe that the holocaust was something only the Nazis are capable of doing.

The survivors had haunting stories to tell. Near starvation was the rule in the camps. The "capo system" coopted inmates into supervisory roles and enforcers of discipline. Their food rations improved with good "service" but resulted in crippling guilt over collaboration with the enemy. Inmates were crowded into unheated facilities and stacked on bunks like cords of wood. Some had to collect hair and gold teeth from the victims of the gas chambers. An Allied bombing raid on a munitions factory near Auschwitz added to their trials. Survival required incredible hardiness and self-control. I wonder if this second "selection" led to the remarkable uniformity amongst the survivors I saw. Most were small, bent by age, reticent, polite, tense and really tough. They also were model citizens. I uncovered not a single case of substance use (which disproves claims about substance use being part of PTSD). None smoked and very few even drank coffee. Many were irritable but none were violent. Almost all worked hard in menial occupations and lived in near poverty. Their complaints were remarkably similar. Nightmares were the rule. They disrupted sleep to the point of sleep deprivation, in itself a health hazard. Many experienced chronic depression, irritability, persistent anxiety, fear of strangers in uniform and had a gloomy outlook.

The assessments were not conducted with later publication in mind. Analysis of data was conducted years later and on the urgings of a colleague. Eventually I published findings on four-hundred-and seventy-four survivors, the first one-hundred-and-twenty-four with the psychologist Brian Cox, the remainder with Neil Rector from CAMH.

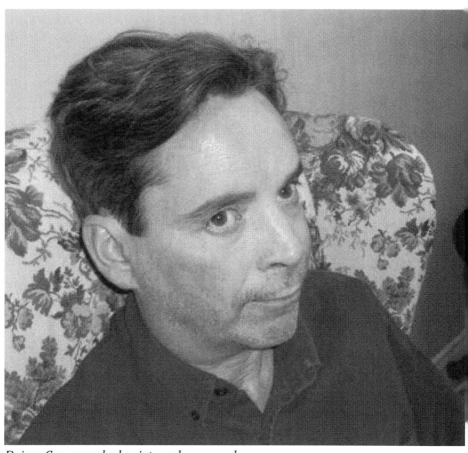

Brian Cox, psychologist and researcher

Both publications compared tattooed Auschwitz survivors with survivors from other camps including Stuthof, Bergen-Belsen, Plaszow, Dachau and Buchenwald. Both have been widely cited in the scientific literature. The first one found that Auschwitz survivors were significantly more impaired than survivors from other camps. It also contained more first claims than the second study. The second study could not replicate this difference between the two groups.

12. Chronic Pain

I must have been a glutton for punishment when adding chronic pain to accidents, assaults and Nazi concentration camps. But, as Oscar Wilde put it so nicely, "I can resist anything but temptation." I couldn't resist when the surgeon Ray Evans invited me to join the Smythe Pain Clinic at Toronto General Hospital. Ray had founded it and made it into the first multi-disciplinary pain clinic in Canada. Its original mandate was cancer pain. Then its focus widened to include chronic pain, the kind of pain that's all over your body and lacks a demonstrable cause.

His clinic brought together four specialties, surgery, neurology, anesthesia and psychiatry. Simple practicality was one reason for this, research the other.

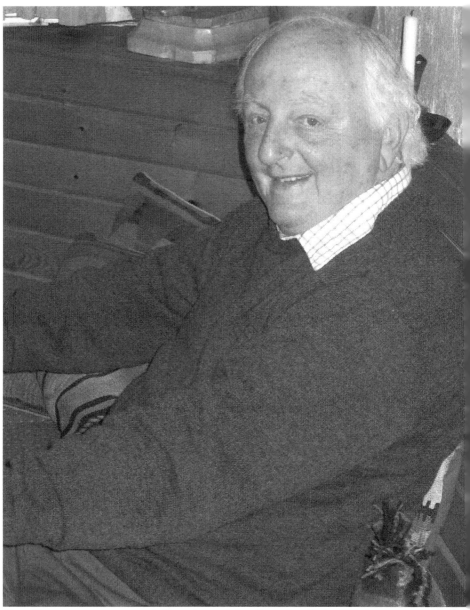

Ray Evans, surgeon and director of the Smythe Pain Clinic

Specialists in solo practice communicate mostly in writing and little time is taken for further discussion with the referral source afterwards. That's a slow way to solve a puzzle like chronic pain.

At the Pain Clinic all specialists shared one single clinical record and practiced in adjacent offices. You could just pop down the hallway if something needed a going-over. The arrangement also eliminated the temptation to view a puzzling case as falling into another specialty's area of responsibility.

Chronic pain is misery plain and simple. There are no smiles, although you meet some of the kindest people there. Typically it's "pain all over", usually affecting muscles and connective tissues. It's also a puzzle by definition. Routine workups are usually complete and analgesics have been tried to the limit. But the pain doesn't let up and there are no obvious leads that tell you what to do (as in the headaches I mentioned earlier).

Accidents commonly start the slide into chronic pain. Later pain location no longer reflects the nature of the accident, a phenomenon that we observed in over a thousand cases. Disability can look dubious, considering that most pain patients don't look all that sick. Tempers flare when a patient feels silently accused of symptom aggravation or worse, particularly in the context of disability and compensation.

More recently a small part of the puzzle has been resolved. Polymyalgia rheumatica has been broken out from chronic pain as a distinct disorder that can be treated effectively with potent anti-inflammatories. Fibromyalgia remained a mystery last time I looked.

Did delusions of competence mislead me into signing up? A very steep learning curve was required. I witnessed physical examinations and picked brains whenever possible. Ray entered patient data into a database during long evenings after work. Databases were an important novelty at the time, enabling us to see the forest beyond the trees. His data enabled statistical evaluation of patient characteristics in regards to demographics and symptoms. It disposed of prejudice such as the "Mediterranean back," a false belief about a tendency of people of Southern origin to dramatize their back complaints.

Additional pieces of the forest began to emerge when our neurologist, Peter Watson, published a study on treating post-herpetic neuralgia with amitriptyline. It was a first in this field.

Connie Bubela, our anesthesiologist, had some success with nerve blocks. The TG Hospital pharmacy was indispensable with its own extensive database on adverse drug reactions and drug-on-drug interactions. These contribute to patients' complaints and were common amongst a clientele that used a multitude of remedies and medications.

Interesting as this was, it still begged the question of how a psychiatrist could function at a pain clinic. Patients also questioned the idea that their pain might have anything to do with psychiatry. As the psychiatrist Howard Merskey remarked: "Pain is pain." Chronic pain is not imaginary and not just "in your mind," even when its cause is hidden. Its experience is a complex process, one that needs explaining.

Lay people picture pain as similar to a phone call. An injury sends a warning signal along a sensory nerve to the brain. The signal includes detail about pain quality (burning, tearing, nagging), about severity and location. That's not the whole story. Research has demonstrated two feedback mechanisms that modulate this incoming signal. The first one is endorphin, the body's own pain reliever. Injury releases it. Conceivably, persistent pain may exhaust its supply. The second feedback mechanism is neural. Ronald Melzack's from the Allan Memorial described it as a "gate" that dampens pain signals as they travel to the brain. His research led to the development of a "dorsal column stimulator" by the neurosurgeon Ron Tasker in Toronto. It's implanted next to the dorsal column of the spine and produces a blocking stimulus that closes Melzack's gate at the push of a button.

Pain becomes intractable and eventually "chronic" when it hits a vulnerable client, one predisposed to suffer complications (in legal lingo a "thin-skulled client). The clients I saw had moved into this stage. All I could do was focus on damage control. I attempted to relieve sleeplessness and depression with antidepressants. Results were mixed. I educated patients about the half-life of drugs, essential to the understanding of break-through pain that develops after half or more of an analgesic dose has been eliminated from the bloodstream. I discussed drug side effects like constipation, sedation and mood change. I looked for drug incompatibilities. A remarkable number of patients remained on medications that seemed useful at one point but created a toxic brew later when combined with others. A combination of ten different medications was pretty much the rule. More was not unusual. Changing doctors and doctor shopping can lead to this level of irrational medication use, also doctors prescribing new drugs without discontinuing the old. Use of multiple pharmacies aggravates the problem further. One single dispenser can spot incompatibilities. Multiple dispensers can't. And people like to hang on to old drugs, just in case. Consequently I asked every new referral to present all pills for inspection, including herbal remedies. One standout turned up with two full shopping bags. He took his pills according to the way he felt. He had blue-pill days, yellow-pill and red-pill days but no no-pill days. Why do people use something that's only marginally effective and not exactly cheap? Excruciating pain carries an intense emotional message: It puts pressure on the doctor to prescribe. She can't just "sit back and do nothing." And giving up on an ineffective medication is easier said than done. "Maybe it helped just a little bit. Maybe pain will worsen without it." And stopping a drug is often easier said than done. Drugs that fail to ease pain can still cause withdrawal symptoms. My efforts rarely got anyone off opiates. But they weren't a total loss. Quite a few habitués ended up with fewer meds, fewer drug interactions and fewer side effects, a small success of sorts.

The current opiate crises resulted from (alleged) over-promotion of opiates and the proverbial swing of the pendulum. It swung from an over-concern about a risk of addiction in cancer to a lack of caution in chronic pain. It's swinging back now. Bringing it to a halt somewhere near an evidence-based middle will require cool heads, diagnostic rigor and more research into the physiology and pharmacology of pain. I would also love to see an end to the uncritical advertisement of over-the-counter analgesics on TV. It's malpractice by media. Drugs are not like soap powder where everyone knows what to expect.

And not all is helpful that's advertised as helpful by glowing testimonials.

Remember: Chronic pain runs an up-and-down course that "regresses towards the mean" (averages out over time). Patients seek help when they feel worse and tend to consider a useless therapy helpful when they get better. One surgeon described this phenomenon as "pills, pulls and the passage of time," with an emphasis on time. Headaches come and go, with or without treatment. So do low back pain, rheumatic pain, anxiety and depression. That's their nature. Advertisements and false promises don't ask this one crucial question: Was it the treatment that helped? Or did pain improve regardless of treatment, just by waiting for a while?

If you find all this rather complicated, there's more to know. The psychologist Wilbur Fordyce was looking for a new way to understand chronic pain. He distinguished between two aspects of it. One aspect is "pain as a private experience." It cannot be observed directly (unless you have access to "evoked potentials" on an EEG). The other aspect is "pain behavior." It can be observed and analyzed. Here's the picture: Suppose a hiker pulls a muscle. She has two choices. She can rest and she can keep on hiking. Lets assume that she ignores her pain and keeps on hiking. A second hiker also pulls a muscle. Lets assume he quits and catches a ride home. Why the difference? Is his pain more severe than hers? We can't know. But we do know that people with similar injuries behave in different ways. And pain behavior has consequences down the road.

In addition to his focus on pain behavior, Fordyce also discriminated between (physical) pain and suffering. Suffering is worrying about the future and what it may bring. Perhaps one of our hikers worried about aggravating his injury. He suffered more and that's why he quit. Perhaps the other one wasn't worried. She suffered less and that's why she didn't quit. In our thought experiment different expectations produce different behaviors. That's a reality that doctors have to manage. Tell your patient that exercise will aggravate his knee and he may become inactive. Tell him that exercise within reason is harmless and he

will keep going. Fordyce's pain clinic in Oregon also managed expectations in a different scenario, when associated with opiate withdrawal. His program reduced opiate doses "blindly." Patients knew neither the timing nor the rate of withdrawal. Identical quantities of syrup disguised the declining doses dissolved in it. Opiates could thus be withdrawn without creating negative expectations at each step.
And there's still more.

We can't measure pain directly. That's a huge disadvantage. Without measurement we are flying blind. But wait a minute. There is a solution. We can measure complaints. The Pain Clinic did this by handing out a brief questionnaire before appointments. It asked patients to darken painful areas with a pen within a silhouette of the frontal and dorsal aspects of the human body. It also asked them to add an estimate of severity (0-10), about effects on sleep, about what helped and what didn't. I added a question about the frequency of pain (as a percentage of waking hours spent in pain). I also assessed the impact of pain on daily living and key activities, screened for anxiety and depression. Why ask all these questions? I was looking for anything that might offer a chance for better damage control. Mood is the lens through which we view reality. When we feel low we expect the worst. When we feel happy we expect better and cope better. Analysis of research data revealed that relentless pain correlated with depressed mood and depressed mood correlated with greater impact of pain on daily living and employment. In other words, when we feel down we become less active physically, socially and vocationally. And when we hit bottom we risk economic hardship. Unrelenting pain plus depression can be the perfect storm. And that's still not all.

When I was a student some rotter threw me off the mat in judo. My neck became stiff and sore. An orthopedic surgeon diagnosed a hairline fracture at a cervical vertebra, prescribed a restraining collar and rest. I followed his advice and got better. Neck pain recurred years later. One arm became partially paralyzed. Eventually this paralysis resolved. Pain improved initially. Then it recurred, lasting several months each time. Painkillers and muscle relaxants proved useless and I stopped them. Traction with a portable unit helped whenever neck spasms threatened. I took my portable traction unit to work and scheduled breaks for its use, keeping well out of the danger zone. The breaks helped me maintain a full schedule. My point is this: I couldn't have done this on a job where taking breaks are impossible. "Disablement" (as some physiotherapists call this) is a process that may accelerate if your job prevents you from listening to your body and from taking breaks when necessary. And once you are on disability you lose endurance and skills.

With chronic pain there are wheels within wheels. You need to practice damage control, listen to your body, be patient and let the pain burn itself out. Preserving sleep, keeping a positive outlook, coping and staying active are crucial. Help from employers can make a big difference, as an exhaustive review of pain studies indicates. It can sometimes right the ship even in a perfect storm.

13. Research

According to the Department of Health total US health care spending reached 3.3 trillion dollars in 2018. That is a lot of cash. That's also a lot of trust. "It works. I tried it," your friends might say about a remedy. But does it really? "In God we trust. All others pay cash" used to read one Florida bumper sticker. That's not a bad idea. Read "testing" for "cash" and it's applicable to health care. FDA- and Health Canada-approved remedies have been tested prior to their release for safety and efficacy. Drugs and supplements not listed on their search pages may not have been tested to the same standards. Just like drugs, health professionals are also tested, regulated and licensed by their respective Boards. Unregulated and unlicensed therapists aren't and may have no adequate training and skills. Scientific-sounding language may disguise this deficiency. I don't know what share of health care dollars snake oils and quackery manage to attract. But I do believe that there's a story to be told. All I can do here is describe what it takes to test a drug for safety and efficacy according to FDA-approved standards. A more general note on junk science might help before we go there. Crucially, science is "not just another opinion" as someone once told me. Science is anything but an opinion. It's a method of testing an opinion. Claims of something "working" are only as reliable as the method that tested them. Scientists' opinions may change. Their methods and testing procedures stay largely constant. So does their habitual caution. Scientists describe their findings in terms of probability, not certainty. Junk science claims certainty. Science papers undergo a peer review before publication to determine if a paper makes the grade. Junk science does not assume these burdens. Some false claims do get published, like the one that claimed a connection between immunization and autism. The paper was withdrawn later, but only after it mislead many. Still, the scientific method is the best we have. Instead of blindly distrusting "school medicine," doubters should ask hard-nosed questions about how an opinion was developed. There are good books on the subject in a wider sense, like Daniel Levitin's "Field Guide To Lies."

Pathology was my first tutor in scientific methodology. In psychiatry I lacked equivalent skills. And then I got lucky. I was invited to participate in the trial of a new anxiolytic benzodiazepine. Participation offered hands-on training and an opportunity to learn from accomplished colleagues. We were to investigate the efficacy of Xanax (Alprazolam) in the treatment of "panic disorder and agoraphobia." I doubted the utility of drug therapy for agoraphobia, but was proven wrong. A study by Donald Klein demonstrated that the antidepressant Imipramine can help. Xanax promised the same benefits as Imipramine, but more quickly and with fewer side effects. Open-label (uncontrolled) phase I studies promised good results. Now Xanax needed a controlled phase II study with a large number of patient-volunteers before the FDA and Canada Health would license its use. Thus began a time I still count as one of the most exiting in my professional life.

There "really is a Kalamazoo" asserted a T-shirt when I arrived at the local airport. Some fifteen other researchers also arrived, to discuss research design and the characteristics of the new drug. They came from Boston, New York, Montreal, Charleston and Toronto. Upjohn, maker of Xanax had taken great care to organize the trial and attract the necessary talent. The company owned a large property in the countryside near the Kellogg Forest, more resort than industrial site. This was the place for our first meeting, with several more to follow. The site included sleeping quarters, conference rooms and a gym, a dining room with top chefs, a book of recipes as a take-home gift and a well-stocked wine cellar. Ponds were stocked with trout. Fishing rods seemed to be waiting for the likes of me near waterside benches, or so I thought. As it turned out, there was no time for fishing or sitting about. Upjohn-issue alarm clocks summoned us to meetings at six every morning. Training sessions lasted the entire day and lunch was brief. Dinner was sumptuous and offered time to compare notes and for light relief. I am most grateful to Jim Ballenger, Chair of the North Carolina department, for his instructions on how to use beer bottle caps as Frisbees.

The Xanax study followed a classical "double-blind placebo-controlled" design. Neither volunteer nor assessor was allowed to know who was on the real drug and who was on the fake pill. Volunteers would have to experience "panic anxiety" (the frights, if you ask me) at least once a week to be enrolled. They would have to discontinue all medications two weeks before the actual trial and remain free of caffeine and alcohol. Assignment to placebo or Xanax was going to be random (by chance). Periodic assessment would evaluate volunteers' mood, anxiety, ability and drug side effects. Our training sessions rehearsed related assessments. They also included diagnostic exercises with videotaped interviews and rehearsal of a standardized interview, the SCID (structured clinical interview according to

DSM). The SCID asked the assessor to read previously validated questions of a page. Most of us found this hard. We were used to asking our own questions and exercise our own judgment. But the SCID had been shown to be more reliable in previous trials than unstructured interviewing and improved agreement between diagnosticians. Assessors also practiced the use of the psychological tests that would be used over the duration of the eight-week study. After a week of rehearsals and brainstorming I returned to Toronto, tired but elated.

A second set of training sessions followed at Massachusetts General Hospital with live patient-volunteers, later a third at the Allan Memorial in Montreal (in connection with another drug trial). – In hindsight this was invaluable, clinically and for legal purposes. It also gave me an inside look into what it's like to do drug research.

Drug trials cost millions of dollars. Potential financial benefits and risks are enormous, as is the pressure on corporate staff, clinical assessors and monitors of procedure. Physician-assessors have to enroll the necessary number of volunteers, follow them up and keep them involved. Too many dropouts would jeopardize reliability and conclusions. Monitors have to ensure that procedures are followed to the T. Statisticians have to crunch the numbers and examine them for levels of significance. Finally, lead investigators describe the method and procedure of the trial, its findings and conclusions in papers submitted to a scientific journal for peer review. Departments of Health review and approve the lot before the drug can be sold in pharmacies.

It's no surprise that it can get hot in the kitchen.

Our share of the first Xanax trial took place at Toronto General Hospital (TGH, part of the University Health Network). Headquarters were at Massachusetts General Hospital. Data collection was stringent. Roving quality-assurance-teams from Upjohn and the FDA monitored data quality at all sites. Some of their visits felt like the FBI had arrived in search of crime. Earlier my friend and colleague Richard Swinson and I had launched the

Anxiety Disorders Clinic at TGH. A press release and additional publicity had increased its visibility.

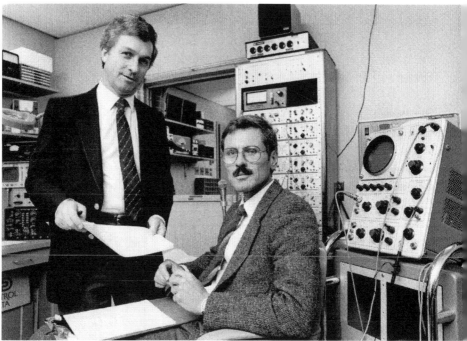

Richard Swinson (left) and the author opening the Anxiety Disorders Clinic at TGH. Getty Images

Potential volunteers still asked many questions before agreeing to participate. This changed after a few TV interviews, which was convenient but also cautionary. It demonstrated that seeing something on TV can be more convincing than it should be. Panickers can get better without drugs. Over a two-week washout period before the actual trial almost one-quarter dropped out. Their symptoms had improved to such an extent that they no longer qualified for participation in the study. Explanations of the nature of panic anxiety may have helped them. Abstention from alcohol and caffeine may have made a difference as well. Upon completion of the trial, data analysis compared Xanax with placebo. Panic frequency was the main criterion. As a group, our volunteers had improved "significantly" and remained improved for as long as they were on Xanax. It seemed at first that we had achieved a break-through. Then doubts developed.

Most family doctors will confirm that only a few of their patients are diagnostically as "pure" as our volunteers. This raises an important question. To what extent can treatment results from a pure sample like ours predict what will happen with real-life patients that suffer from several different ailments? Questions from skeptical GPs reinforced my own doubts, as did a comment by the British psychiatrist Isaac Marks who "would love to do a trial with volunteers who failed entrance criteria." The first Xanax trial also did not tell us how patients would manage after Xanax is withdrawn. A second trial at the Toronto and Montreal sites examined this and was as discouraging as the first study was encouraging. All volunteers completed their withdrawal. That was the good news. The bad news was that all relapsed. Some were worse off than before. To their credit, Upjohn agreed to fund a third Xanax trial. It compared the benefits of Xanax with therapist-assisted exposure therapy (behavior therapy). This trial became known as the London-Toronto study. It deserves detailed mention as it was (and probably still is) the largest such study published on the treatment of agoraphobia.

Study design was again of the classical double blind placebo controlled variety. But this time, volunteers were randomly subdivided into four subgroups: Xanax/placebo-exposure, Xanax/exposure, drug-placebo/exposure and drug-placebo/placebo-exposure. The placebo-exposure groups received relaxation training. The drug-placebo groups received a fake pill. Also new was a six-month follow-up that required abstinence from further treatment. It was added to determine long-term treatment outcome. Our results were unpopular with Upjohn. As in the two preceding studies, volunteers on Alprazolam improved rapidly. As in the previous withdrawal study, they lost their improvement on withdrawal. Exposure therapy (desensitization) on its own resulted in slow but persistent improvement that continued during follow-up. The exposure group fared best. Relaxation training did not help.

Xanax/exposure also did not lead to lasting improvement. The bottom line was clear: Behavior therapy yielded better results than Xanax and worked better without Xanax as an add-on. These findings were aired in the august setting of a Geneva conference room and created a great deal of heat, some of it in a language I have never before or since heard in a meeting of scientists. Fortunately it reached eight ears only. I am unaware of any support from Upjohn to disseminate the results. But published they were. A subsequent exchange of Letters to the Editor in the British Journal of Psychiatry documents a controversy that continued for some time. I signed one of the letters authored by Isaac Marks, the British lead investigator and a highly respected researcher. It's dry and to the point: "Scientific research and marketing are two separate disciplines." They should not be intermingled.

I don't believe that the London/Toronto study damaged Upjohn's financial interests. Xanax remains one of the most prescribed benzodiazepines, although its use has been eclipsed by SSRI antidepressants. I take off my hat to the volunteers who made the London-Toronto study possible, particularly their compliance with the six-month follow-up that had to be endured without further treatment. Which brings me to another issue: They were members of the public. It stands to reason that research data harvested with help from the public should be in the public domain, including disappointing results. And, as detective Colombo was fond of saying, there's "one more thing:" Drug efficacy is usually reported as (statistically) "significant." Significant efficacy is not equivalent to "clinical effectiveness." It reflects a statistic finding, not proof of a worthwhile health benefit. For that "clinical effectiveness" is better. It has been defined as a reduction of symptoms by some 50%. At that level daily life really does get better. At a lesser level that may not be the case. Drug trials should make these findings available to prescribing physicians.

To provide some examples: Certain medications for the heart, antibiotics, antipsychotics and a number of psychiatric drugs easily rise to the 50% benchmark. But they do so only when used for the correct indications, for the correct length of time and in the correct dosage. Used haphazardly they can fool with users' body chemistry just like street drugs do.

What's the bottom line to our Xanax trial? I am not advising against drug trials or participation in them, no matter how critical all the above may sound. Quite the opposite. Well-researched treatments are safer and more reliable than treatments that are untested. Scientific research tells you what you are getting. Volunteers can also benefit from participation. Well-designed trials may offer a more thorough assessment and closer follow-up than clinical practice. And volunteers get a chance to try the latest treatment that wouldn't be available elsewhere. For myself, I wouldn't miss participation in the Xanax trials for anything. It sharpened my skills, facilitated my own research and improved my medico-legal work.

Onwards to an entirely different subject, the car accidents I mentioned earlier. Roughly 7 million car accidents happen annually in the US. The US Department of Transportation reports their combined costs as 242 billion dollars for 2010. Again, that's a lot of cash. That's also a lot of pain, suffering and litigation. What happens to survivors of car accidents after the dust has settled? A substantial percentage suffers from injuries for years to come. Some of their injuries are invisible as an analysis of Canadian data found and more impaired than their visible injuries suggest.

A Toronto surgeon had a go at seemingly "psychosomatic" neck pain after car accidents. Experiments with monkeys identified one culprit, a hyperextension injury that rear-end impact can cause when poorly designed car seats have a headrest that's too low. And there is a second invisible injury that changes lives and causes economic damage. As described earlier, survivors of car accidents may develop symptoms of PTSD. Now to the million-dollar research question: Are accidents really to blame for these phobias or were these people phobic anyway? Experiments with volunteers were not an option. Richard Swinson and I looked for a symptom cluster that was as unique as a fingerprint and characteristic for accident survivors with PTSD. And we found one: They all had the frights, feared accidents, had nightmares of accidents and were excessively security-conscious. They also had not been anxious before their accident. And, to top it all off, a sizeable percentage improved with exposure to riding in cars. Focusing on the most relevant characteristic, I christened their phobia "accident phobia."

My observations had taken place over ten years, starting in the mid-seventies. I might have never published the results, a "first" in the medical literature as it turned out, had Richard Swinson not encouraged me. Publication wasn't easy. Nobody believes readily in something completely new that implies a common liability. Two journals rejected our manuscript and a third, the Canadian Journal of Psychiatry accepted it only after a very lengthy review. Publication then set a process in motion that led to the development of a treatment manual published by the American Psychological Association and to the development of a brief questionnaire (the Accident Fear Questionnaire) together with Brian Cox. The AFQ explores characteristic complaints and behavior change after MVA and takes only five minutes to complete. Before publication it went through a validation process. That compared the results of a separate assessment for PTSD with the results of the AFQ. They matched. Most importantly, women were not over-represented as they usually are in case of spontaneously emerging phobias. Another finding is also of interest here. Behavioral data (changes in driving habits) were more reliable predictors of PTSD than patients' complaints.

Some research does not require volunteers, experimentation or systematic clinical observation like the research described above. One is meta-analysis that combines existing data from several trials and re-analyzes them. The psychologist Steven Taylor masterminded one such study. He re-analyzed data from two different populations with PTSD, one set from Canadian peacekeepers and one from survivors of car accidents. "Core symptoms" of PTSD were remarkably similar for both groups, suggesting that a well-defined set of characteristics describes full-fledged PTSD from any cause. This bolsters the standing of PTSD as a valid psychiatric diagnosis.

Another literature study concerned itself with chronic pain. How valid is it as a concept and as a diagnosis? Chronic pain is remarkably common. According to NIH (The National Institute for Complementary and Integrative Health) close to 20% of US adults had chronic pain and some 8% had "high-impact pain" (the kind that became the focus of the Pain Clinic). Prevalence was similar both in Canada and in a European survey. This and concerns over health care funding inspired a systematic review of the entire scientific literature on chronic pain, a massive task. "Systematic" meant that criteria for including a scientific paper in the final analysis were pre-determined before librarians began the initial literature search. They included only peer-reviewed publications for further review and only studies that followed their subjects longitudinally (going forward over time). The Government of Ontario, the Ministry of Health and Welfare and the Workers Safety and Insurance Board sponsored the project. A team of statisticians evaluated the data collated by the librarians. A committee of specialists reviewed and summarized them subject-by-subject. It was multi-disciplinary and included a neurosurgeon, an orthopedic surgeon, a physiatrist, a physiotherapist, an occupational therapist, a chiropractor and myself. (And I probably forgot someone.) We discussed an enormous amount of evidence. The Clinical Journal of Pain published the resulting monograph in 2001. It reaffirmed chronic pain as a valid health issue and summarized promising interventions. It was gratifying to see that it also influenced Ontario health policy.

14. The Rubber Chicken Circuit

Standing at a podium in Montreal's big arena was nerve-racking. The auditorium held close to three thousand. Looking down from a dizzying height, I could believe it. The place was buzzing.

People were chatting, moving seats, walking in and out. It was a public forum on anxiety and I felt like a clinical example of it when my turn came to utter a few introductory words. I began with two or three stock French sentences. That didn't turn any heads. Maybe Montrealers are bored with sycophants. I switched to English with a personal story about a long-departed aunt proverbial for her terror of missing a train. My disconnect with the crowd continued. Thankfully another speaker took over after the allotted five minutes. He got a similar reception. The audience finally came to life during the question-and-answer part of the forum. Then questions came thick and fast. It almost felt like fun. After it was all over our corporate sponsors rewarded us with a non-Clintonesque sum.

After the launch of the Anxiety Disorders Clinic requests to participate in forums, shows and roundtables trickled in. Most shows were phone-ins on the radio. It was hard to connect with an audience when nobody was in the room. TV was easier. I could look at the host and the facial expressions of the studio crew to get feedback, but risked only the occasional sideways glance. More might look shifty. Coaches tell you to make love to the camera. I imagined the caller's face inside the lens and talk to it as if in conversation. There never was much back-and forth. One reply to a question was it. Then we moved to the next call in the line-up. Humor could be toxic. When a moderator wasn't present it got lonely. Once I was led to a cubbyhole in the CBC's old TV studio on Yonge Street. Cardboard boxes lined the wall. A camera pointed at my face. And that was it. The moderator was in Alberta. Presumably a picture of Toronto was inserted behind my back. A picture of the boxes would have been more honest. A light came on once we were live. I was told that millions watched the show (probably while eating lunch). I should have waved.

Publicity does have its rewards though. An unexpected one came in the shape of a phone call. Leonard Nemoy of "Star Wars" fame wanted my office for a movie with a psychiatric theme. He was directing, "The Good Mother." Dianne Keaton played the lead. Was someone pulling my leg? I asked a few questions and agreed. How could I not? Gargantuan trucks pulled up on the appointed days for the stars to hide in. I met the famous one and the lime-lights came on. The "psychiatrist" in the picture looked like the villain of the plot, cold and devoid of empathy. I had facilitated my own symbolic hanging. But watching it unfold was exiting and it paid. Another reward came from Myers Briggs, a drug company. Myers Briggs hosted a visit to their research facility in Wallingford, New Jersey. They were researching "lazarones," a new class of agents intended to resurrect dying tissue after strokes and heart attacks on hamster brains (sorry, no news to date). Research data were closely held to prevent unwanted transfer of proprietary knowledge. Staff was not allowed to take any written information outside the building. They hadn't lost their sense of humor though, labeling their presentation "pharmaco-theatre." Myers Briggs also made Buspirone, a non-sedating tranquillizer potentially useful to anxious people who had to be alert enough to operate machinery and react quickly in emergencies. This seemed medically useful. It also interested the US Army. Front-line troops may "freeze" in terror when faced with a mortal threat. Some time after my visit a US Army officer turned up in his civvies at Anxiety Disorders to pick Richard's and my brains. He might as well have turned up in uniform, with his razor-sharp crease in his trousers and boots polished to a shine. But I liked him, laid back as he was just like my former supervisor at the VA and a medical author in his own right. Nothing came of the visit.

This was the big time, if you want to call it that. The rest was more down-market.
I volunteered for talks to the general public on anxiety disorder and phobias. Few people trickled into these small seminars and most sat as far as from the speaker as possible. An early partner was a Toronto psychologist named Quirk. Introduced as "Kook & Quirk" we extolled on the merits of behavior therapy and systematic desensitization. The Ministry of Health sponsored a few seminars on pain. For these I joined Ray Evans from the Pain Clinic. The seminars were clinical discussion groups with doctors and nurses in remote communities. Sometimes it

seemed the local doctors had beaten the bushes for the hardest cases with the most vexing diseases, guaranteed to stump the bigwigs from Toronto. When stumped, admit it and commiserate. There was also a lot to admire in rural practice, dedication, grit and managing with small resources. Two drug companies sponsored unpaid talks about medications. For Upjohn it was Xanax. Their requests dried up after the dustup in Geneva. Next came Myers Briggs and their drug Buspirone. The routine was always the same. A rep would pick me up in Toronto and drive me to a small community where a few GPs would attend my dog-and-pony show, encouraged by a promise of supper and a bit of socializing. I saw places I would have never visited otherwise. Unforgettable was a drive into an incredibly long sunset under a fall sky in the northern prairies. Bales of straw stood out like torches while the stubble was already in the shadows. One GP took me to a fur traders' warehouse in Ontario's north. It was filled with rich pelts from wolves, bears, caribou and beaver. Other GPs had stories to tell. How many cars does it take on a cold winter day to fog in an intersection in South Porcupine? - Only two. How does one land a plane on a frozen lake when a snow-white surface blends in with a white horizon? – Very, very gently. And what is the most common traffic accident in parts of Ontario's North? - Moose against snowmobile.

Doctors in remote communities cope with massive workloads and little reprieve. They cover call for each other and socialize together. Being single is hard. Doctors are not allowed to date their patients, past or present. That leaves few options. In the resigned words of one, "I'd have to thumb it on the highway or surf the Internet." Supper was very well done chicken, its deep-fried relation or local fare. I became expert on anything melted onto toast and discovered chicken fingers, if there's such a thing. But the circuit got me out of the office and widened my horizons. I learned as much as I taught about medications in general and the discontinuation of benzodiazepines in particular. Once an entire audience cancelled at short notice for reasons unclear. Arrangements had been costly. On-site advertisement was limited to a display of drugs on a side table. Our arrangement was purer than the driven snow and the sponsor was not amused. Three university-based medical specialists from Toronto had been flown in for a seriously academic meeting on the medical and psychological aspects of stress. Stress and no food or drink? Rumor had it that this omission was the reason for the cancellation. The three of us went ahead anyway and lectured each other. It was my smallest audience ever and one of the most responsive.

Any form of drug advertisement is now *verboten* according to College rules. I still don't regret it, given the experience it provided at the time.

15. Medico-Legals

Most of us like to stay clear of the courts, myself included. They are intimidating places. Lawyers dress in long black gowns, cart about vast stacks of documentation and gather in groups to whisper confidentialities. Judges are rarely seen until they appear in full regalia to calls of "all rise," which we dutifully do. Courtrooms display heraldic symbols that represent the supreme power of the Law. And what happens there changes lives, often permanently. Anyone who doubts that anticipatory anxiety has physical consequences should visit the washrooms at a courthouse. The evidence is there for all to see (and for hapless cleaners to remove). Anyone who fears public speaking and "negative evaluation" is in for a special treat, particularly anyone who functions as an expert witness. A tough cross-examiner has plenty to ask about qualifications, the basis for "your valued opinions" and grasp of the evidence, while skillfully undermining credibility.

My interest in the unholy triad of anxiety, pain and psychological trauma attracted much legal attention. Many "invitations" to testify arrived on my desk. If the plaintiff was also a client of mine, I would send a copy of the relevant medical record to her attorney after receiving a legally binding release. I might also write a covering letter that summarized illness, its causes, treatment and related disability. Or I might refrain from giving any opinion, depending on the case. Usually that was it. Most insurance cases settled out of court. Occasionally a battle between experts ensued before a settlement. Rarely was I summoned to attend court under threat of punishment. If that happened without prior agreement over cost, losses and expenses were my problem.

That's what happened with one summons I received in the middle of winter. I was starved for sun and had a pre-paid vacation to the Caribbean. My pleas for accommodation fell on deaf ears. I contacted the Law Society and declared my willingness to attend at any time whatsoever, except for the one specified by the summons. They were most understanding and had a chat with the issuer of the summons. He wouldn't budge (as was his right). Gnashing my teeth I took a closer look at the hated piece of paper and, eureka, a clerical error had came to my rescue. The summons listed the time of the hearing but not the place. It looked invalid. I checked with someone in the legal fraternity. Reassured, I left for the Caribbean after snail-mailing a letter to counsel, indicating where I might be reached.

Court work teaches you two lessons right off the bat: Read everything and accept as many ups and downs as there are in Raymond Chandler's thriller of "Trouble Is My Business."

Fortunately summonses were rare. One or two were delivered to my home, announced *sotto voce* by the server and intended to rattle my cage. Beyond that, testifying rarely caused problems thanks to counsels' consideration and coverage by helpful colleagues. Opposing counsel could be icily polite in cross-examination, but that was it. "With due respect" was the stock line that preceded even a hint of confrontation. Only once was I faced with an attempt of outright intimidation. It turned into an entertaining moment.

A mother was suing for compensation after a fatal road accident. The amount exceeded the provisions of Family Law. The plaintiff based her excess demand on emotional damages and I was called to testify for the Defense. She was visibly angry and noisily interrupted proceedings at one point. Counsel for Plaintiff took it from there. He approached the witness box where I stood, the villain who dared to cast doubt upon the veracity of his client's claim. His act was flawless. His head was raised high, his gaze piercing. His black gown and long black mane flowed with each step as he approached the witness box. Moving ever closer he fired question after question. He had a reputation and he was confirming it, shouting his last question right into my face just feet away. Up to then I had parsed my responses. Now it was my turn for theatrics. I paused for effect, then asked him quietly if he could "please speak up," barely loud enough for the judge to hear. His Honor smiled ever so slightly. Counsel was not amused. He held aloft a large file, shook it violently and demanded to know if I had read it. My response was flippant enough to invite reproach from his Honor: "Can I wait for the movie?" The crowded courtroom collapsed in laughter and the cross-examination ended shortly afterwards.

Such moments of levity were rare. It's far easier to be the proverbial deer in the headlights, especially as a beginner. When an Alabama psychiatrist was charged with defrauding Medicare, his defense attorney retained me to challenge testimony for the prosecution. The witnesses were former patients of the psychiatrist. FBI agents had interviewed them and asked if they recalled as many visits from the doctor as he had billed for? The patients recalled some visits but not all, apparently confirming the prosecution's charge of excess billing. I questioned the reliability of their memories. All had been on a psychiatric ward during the relevant times and on tranquillizers that impair memory. I cited corroborative reports from an American psychiatric textbook. The cross-examining State attorney seemed to go easy on me. On closing he asked innocently if I was a "friend of the defendant." I said so and left it at that. The judge then disallowed my testimony as "biased" and my friend was convicted.

The ruling of "bias" bothered me for years. I should have pushed back with something like "two plus still make four, even if a friend of the accused says so." I had to learn the ropes. Experience helped some. Then a legal journal advertised a course on cross-examination at Osgood Law School in Toronto. Nobody asked any questions when I registered there together with a colleague. The instructors found us out quickly enough. It didn't matter. Everyone had a good laugh and they let us stay. The course covered the ground rules of roping in a hostile witness. It was important to ask only questions that led to predictable answers, never open-ended ones. If successful, the strategy puts the witness in a bind. He will either have to agree with the cross-examiner or accept the poisoned chalice of contradicting himself. All this should be done without personal denigration. Participants practiced in pairs. The others watched and critiqued. I liked the course so much I took it twice.

Preparing testimony can be tedious. Plaintiffs and defendants must be interviewed meticulously, preferably without losing cooperation in an adversarial situation. Commonly a thousand pages or more of clinical records, police reports and reports from opposing experts require careful review. Sometimes the best bits were in a small scribbled note. All relevant detail has to be integrated into one cohesive picture that includes anything that goes for and against a claim. Is the claim in keeping with clinical experience? Is it in keeping with scientific findings? Is it based on observations that have been independently confirmed? Reports have to be written with close attention to logic and detail and in plain English. Anticipating court was nerve-racking for me, no matter how confident I might feel about my knowledge of the subject. My handiwork and my ability to think on my feet would both be put to the test there.
Discussions with retaining counsel helped greatly. Occasionally it added levity. Before the criminal case against the Alabama psychiatrist I met his defense attorney. He had an elegant office

adjacent to a square in downtown Mobile. My evidence was full of medical terminology. This however was a jury trial and more fitting language was called for. Counsel delivered his advice in a lovely Southern drawl: "Doc," he said, "you must put the hay where the goats can get at it." His trust in local security was as low as it was in the jury's intellect. He holstered his Colt before accompanying me downstairs to a taxi stand.

In preparation to the Ssenjonga case (see below) the Crown attorney delivered another piece of important advice, this one more serious. This case was about sexual transmission of a lethal illness and emotionally charged. Daily newspaper headlines were raising the emotional temperature even further and I was in danger of becoming the white knight riding to the victims' rescue. As we sat in a London sidewalk café he pointed out various passers-by. They included assailants, fraudsters and thieves, some who had been convicted and some that got away. The Law did not dish out "justice" as the public sees it, he said. It does not convict on the basis of moral outrage. It "settles" cases on the basis of admissible evidence. Period. I read this this as a warning: Describe your evidence, matter of fact and carefully. Sometimes though one forgets.

I was working on a defense report in a civil case and I was late. I was also late with an academic paper and my patient load was at critical levels. I had worked through a night and finished my medico-legal report in the early morning hours. I wanted it off my desk and out the door. And somehow in my eagerness, I managed to not proofread three pages. They were full of errors as first drafts often are. All errors were quotes from a file and labeled as such. None were of the kind that alters conclusions. However the plaintiff complained to the College of Physicians and Surgeons of Ontario. It took considerable effort to convince the College investigator that the complaint was over the top. The complainant was not my patient, as he seemed to suggest. My errors were clerical and not material. I had also corrected them once they were queried. And the College investigator was intervening in an ongoing legal case. Crucifixion averted: The complaint was dismissed without a record. But the lesson stuck. I have never sent out a report in a hurry since then and preferably not unless at least one day has passed since its writing.

I also made it my practice to accept work on behalf of both the Defense and the Crown in criminal cases, on behalf of plaintiff and defense in civil cases. This keeps you honest. It can also be risqué. An attorney might remember testimony from an earlier case and use it against me. I was either lucky or my three rules of reporting saved me. They are "describe, describe and then describe some more." Describing means saying what you see, when, where and how you see it and how you arrive at your conclusions. It's the attorney's job to argue the case. Opinions should be parsed. Consequently I have never labeled someone a "fake," no matter how unusual a claim might be.

I testified reluctantly at first, then with increasing ease. At first I refused to testify on behalf of a physician because the prospect made me nervous. He did just fine without my help. Then I refused a high-profile criminal case. It was about a murder committed with elaborate preparation "while sleepwalking." Both refusals felt like a cop-out afterwards. I finally accepted a criminal case about a wrongful conviction (Guy-Paul Morin) when assured that the Appeals Court would receive my written report without requiring oral testimony. Then came the proverbial bolt out of the blue, a formal appointment to German courts concerning "*Wiedergutmaching*" (restitution) to Jewish concentration survivors. This was politically sensitive work, but still not in open court and adversarial. I had the privilege to function as a "Friend of the Court," having to support neither the State nor the plaintiff in these cases. The Ontario Workplace Safety and Insurance Board and its Tribunal required a similarly neutral posture. Eventually my publications on psychological trauma and pain attracted requests to testify in adversarial cases. Fortunately the four criminal cases mentioned below were all right up my alley in anxiety disorders.

In three of the five cases below the defense used "panic" to get their client off the hook. In the fourth the defense used it to exempt a police officer from testifying. In the fifth the Crown relied on an alleged threat to the mental health of the general public to keep videotaped evidence of a murder away from the media. Every one of them tested my mettle.

Guy Paul Morin (Court of Appeal, 1992): Police sergeant M was an identification officer and witness on behalf of the Crown. Cigarette butts had been found near the victim's body, but Morin was a non-smoker. M had kept two notebooks on this case, one for "raw notes" and one that contained the "final version." The raw notes could not be located. The defense was appealing an earlier conviction. It wanted to re-examine M under oath, to explore discrepancies in his evidence.

The Crown resisted this request. Its experts claimed that M suffered from PTSD and from heart disease. He had required coronary bypass surgery and was on antihypertensive medication. A Wechsler Memory Scale found "impaired cognitive function, attributable to stress." Another psychological test, the MMPI, was considered indicative of "somatic delusions." Crucially, the Crown claimed that M might die in court from a heart attack during cross-examination.

The ***Defense*** cardiology expert confirmed high blood pressure. However M had "recovered" from bypass surgery. His pharmacological management was "suboptimal" (polite for "poor") and needed improving. My psychiatric report noted panic anxiety, hyperventilation and driving fears related to a car accident. The presence of delusions could not be confirmed. M's fear of heart attacks was typical for panic anxiety and common in physically healthy panickers. Anxiety did not endanger his life. His medication included Secobarbital. It was indeed "suboptimal." He was able to testify once his doctor prescribed more appropriately.

The **judge** ruled that M would testify in an informal setting. Morin's appeal was rejected. A second appeal included new DNA evidence and Morin was finally exculpated.

Charles Ssenjonga *(1993)* was an AIDS carrier, indicating a condition that was almost always fatal at the time. His physician informed him of the diagnosis. Health authorities ordered him to refrain from unprotected intercourse. In contravention of this order S (allegedly) infected several women with the AIDS virus. They testified that S had not alerted them to his illness before consorting with them and had not used precautions. S suffered from a rare strain of AIDS, which identified him as the source of the victims' infection. By the time he was criminally charged, he was suffering from bacterial infections, fevers and had a skin condition. He wanted to stay out of jail until he died.

The Crown alleged that S had acted in wanton disregard for the victims' health. It sought a precedent-setting conviction.

The **Defense** team stated that S was suffering from PTSD and had therefor been unable to "appreciate" the risk of passing on his HIV virus. His PTSD was attributable to the Ugandan War. S had witnessed Idi Amin's troops beat people there and this "traumatized" him. He was "traumatized" again when his doctor told him he had AIDS. Subsequently he suffered from PTSD between 1989 and 1990. Defense experts offered detailed psychometrics and neuropsychological testing to support their conclusion (none designed to identify PTSD). They claimed that "dissociative phenomena and denial" had rendered S incapable of using proper judgment (an insanity defense based on psychoanalytic theory).

Crown: Detailed examination by Structured Clinical Interview (SCID), the Impact of Events Scale (which quantifies impairment of daily living) and a behavioral assessment were inconsistent with a diagnosis of PTSD. S had experienced panic anxiety (the frights), but only in situations he perceived as confining. He displayed no abnormal fears of AIDS and was capable of discussing AIDS-related topics. He was also active sexually. He did not harbor an abnormal fear of violence (as in PTSD after assault) or an abnormal fear of negative evaluation (as in social anxiety when someone can't say "no"). He merely avoided informing his sexual partners. His current distress was caused by his illness and by the criminal charges he was facing. It was not a sign of psychiatric disorder.

S admitted during my interview that his actions had been "immature." Being criminally charged made him realize that he had "erred." (This evidence was inadmissible in Court). I concluded that the defense theory lacked factual and diagnostic support. And none of the above rendered S incapable of informing his victims that he had AIDS.

During the trial, **Counsel for the defense** conducted a very thorough cross-examination that lasted a day-and-a-half. At one point he suggested that only psychoanalysts could judge matters related to the (Freudian) mechanisms of defense like dissociation and denial. Consequently I (the non-psychoanalyst) wasn't qualified to testify on psychoanalytic findings. I countered that I had read Freud in the German original, while his experts had read him in disputed translation. He pointed out that frequent discussion of AIDS had improved S' ability to discuss it. I pointed out that evidence supporting a diagnosis of PTSD past and present was lacking, that memories like his about school might explain some of his actions as understandable but they did not compel his actions. He had acted willfully.

The **judge** had written some 130 pages of his ruling when S died of unknown causes. His ruling remains undisclosed.

This trial was my baptism of fire. My cross- examiner was well known for his skills and persistence. His cross-examination took far longer and was far more detailed than I had expected. I sweated it, literally and so much that the Crown attorney treated me to a fresh shirt from a nearby supermarket. After the trial the journalist June Callwood published a book titled "Trial without End" (1995). It details S' history but not the clash between psychoanalytic theory and observable evidence that I was to encounter over and over again in other cases.

Appleton (1994) stood accused of having murdered his mother-in-law. She had sustained five bullet wounds from an unrifled and untraceable handgun and some sixty severe blows to her head.

On the night of the murder A's father-in-law returned late from work. He found his spouse in a pool of blood, called 911 and attempted resuscitation. A had been invited for dinner that night but wasn't there when his father-in-law arrived at the scene. A explained his absence by having been late himself. When he finally arrived at his in-laws residence the police were there and he left without going inside. When confronted with blood evidence, he changed his story. He claimed that he had found his bloodied mother-in-law at the scene, tried to revive her, then fled in a "panic." According to witnesses he dumped the floor mats and the mats from the trunk of his car afterwards. He also bought fresh clothing at a Hasty Market and paid with a bloodstained bill (which led to the detectives nick-naming him "Hasty Bill").

The **Defense** explained A's actions in medical terms as "panic (anxiety)." He had feared that the police might frame him for the murder. According to a psychologist and a psychiatrist, his past explained this reaction. He had been "traumatized" at the age of eight when dogs attacked him during an altercation with one of his mother's boyfriends. He was "traumatized" again when he witnessed his father's stroke. These two experiences caused him to "deny" events that "looked wrong." He attempted to "displace" them (an unconscious defense according to psychoanalytic theory) and expected blame for all wrongs no matter how unjustified. He became alcoholic.

A's family believed in his innocence.

The **Crown** retained my colleague Peter Collins as expert witness. I acted in support and did not testify. A refused all interviews. This limited us to a review of the available records. We challenged the credibility of defense reports. A had coped with sights of blood and injury when working at a hospital. He had travelled to London and borrowed a manual on how to build an unrifled firearm (according to Scotland Yard). He exhibited none of the clinical characteristics of (DSM) panic disorder. Defense reports had used the term "panic" in lay terms and not as defined by DSM. In addition, A had offered contradictory testimony and hadn't revealed his two past marriages to his current spouse. His in-laws were affluent (and his spouse could expect a sizeable inheritance). I examined A's financial records and found evidence of unsustainable spending. He had burned a previous partner's clothing (displaying aggression). He had no past history of anxiety or mood disorder, which would portray him as "thin-skulled" (vulnerable). He sounded calm on police surveillance tapes, once speaking of wearing "brothel creepers"

(English slang for crepe-soled shoes) that made detectives wonder if they had uncovered a sex ring. A became distressed only later, after he had been charged with murder. Most importantly, he revealed details about the murder to the defense psychiatrist that only the murderer could have known. A was convicted of murder and sentenced to life.

Paul Bernardo (1995) had videotaped several of his murderous sexual assaults. Once discovered and surrendered by his attorney, the tapes became crucial evidence. They depict Bernardo and his partner Karla Homulka during the rape and the systematic humiliation of two victims. Two police detectives reviewed the tapes and suffered considerable distress as a consequence. Bernardo's trial was front-page news and included horrendous details. The families of the victims complained of severe distress over this publicity and wanted the videotapes permanently sealed. Their complaint became the focus of a separate hearing. The **Crown** argued for a ban, to accommodate the families' and to protect the general public from psychological harm unrestricted publication might cause. The **Media** objected and obtained Intervener status. They argued for full public access to the evidence. A ban would interfere with free speech and the public's "right to know."

Experts for the **Crown** claimed that victims' families would have no choice but to attend court. Public display of the videos "would repeat the assaults in their mind" and aggravate the psychiatric condition experienced by some of them. Public access might also trigger psychiatric conditions in "Jane Doe" (the public). This was likely as the media had been "grossly insensitive" to date.

Counsels for the Media argued that their right to free speech was guaranteed by the Constitution. They retained three psychiatric experts (including myself) who prepared separate reports. The reports stated that heinous crimes were routinely discussed in court and that obscenity laws already restricted publication. Admittedly, the videotapes would be distressing to almost anyone. They could also be "cathartic," even "educational" to the public as exemplified by a British murder case. The police detectives however had no other choice but to pay close attention to every single detail on the tapes. Victims' families and the general public did have this choice. They were free not to attend court and free to avert their eyes if attending. The physicians arguing against publication were over-reaching. Instead of arguing against freedom of speech and the public's right to know they should discourage attendance by anyone whose health they considered endangered.

Justice Lesage was going to allow the audiotaped portion of the murder evidence into open court while limiting the visual material to judge, jury and defendant. Upon appeal, the **Supreme Court of Canada** let the ruling stand.

Patrick Kelly (Court of Appeal, 1998) was a colorful undercover RCMP drug squad officer who had been convicted of murder in 1984. He had thrown his wife from a high-rise balcony at Palace Pier in Toronto. Injuries from the fall had obscured any signs of a struggle. K claimed that it had been an accident. However his ex-girlfriend T testified that she had witnessed the murder. She had been a close friend of the victim. She did not come forward for several years, explaining this delay as "trying to block the murder from her mind." K was convicted on the basis of her eyewitness testimony. "The Judas Kiss" by M. Harris (1995) publicized the case.

In 1998 T recanted. She now claimed that she had not witnessed the murder. She also lodged a complaint against the police psychiatrist who had taken her original deposition together with two detectives. She claimed that he had "hypnotized" her. And now she had realized that her memory and her original deposition had been "a dream." She realized this while "panicking" on top of a high tower.

K appealed his earlier conviction on the grounds of this recantation. This made his appeal a psychiatric case and the first such case before the Court of Appeals since the Sixties. It was precedent setting.

His **Defense** argued that T's recantation presented new and credible evidence.

The **Crown** argued that her recantation was fictitious. Unfortunately T had moved abroad and was unavailable for re-examination. I was retained to review the file.

T had been in psychological treatment for anxiety disorder and possibly for PTSD. She did fear heights. She had been assaulted before and after the murder and had been in a car crash. (Both may cause PTSD.) However her claim of erroneous testimony due to false memory was unverifiable and unlikely. I had never come across a case before where someone recognized a memory as "false" while "panicking." In fact, the scientific literature reports that traumatic memories are unforgettable and difficult to dismiss.

My testimony was unopposed. The appeal failed.

A **criminal rape case** against former Nova Scotia premier **Gerald Regan (2002)** was heard in camera under a publication ban. I testified on behalf of the **Defense**. Invisible and unverifiable mental processes were an issue once again. – Regan was found not guilty.

In one murder case my expertise was subjected to an unusual challenge. The defendant had previously claimed "conversion" blindness in an unrelated matter. Questions arose regarding his credibility. Counsel for the Defense

questioned my qualification to testify, which is routine. Then he asked if I had ever seen a case of "conversion blindness." I hadn't and said so (failing to include "credible"). Counsel then claimed I was "not qualified, as I had no experience in the matter." I was annoyed by what looked like a ruse and asked if I could tell him a little story. Mistakenly he agreed. I made one up on the fly about an old farmer who was asked if he knew any flying cows. The farmer answered no, he had never seen one. I then suggested that, according to counsel's logic, this farmer didn't know cows. – His Honor qualified me. Counsel gave me a very dirty look.

One newspaper report cited the psychologist Steven Taylor on a similar case. With bull's-eye accuracy he called such unverifiable theories "cognitive science fiction."

Policing can be stressful to say the least. Under-cover officers have to assume a criminal identity and risk their lives if outed. Officers walking the beat risk dog bites, assaults and being swarmed. They have to approach dangerous suspects and may find themselves looking into the muzzle of a gun. A degree of edginess must be expected in anyone who works under such circumstances. Legal issues arise when edginess morphs into over-reaction and violence. Courts have to determine in such cases if unlawful acts were willful or a consequence of psychiatric illness. Two criminal trials of police officers resembled the five cases described above in regards to their defense. The first case was about spousal abuse, the second about fraud. Neither officer met diagnostic criteria for a psychiatric disorder.

Instead of repeating much of the above, a fictitious cross-examination of an equally fictitious expert may summarize my challenge of a defense based on unverifiable theory.

"Counsel: If I understand you correctly, you are saying that repression of an unacceptable event occurred in this case and that this repressed memory affected the conduct of the defendant. Expert: Yes, I understand that that's what happened. Counsel: Please help me understand the process of repression. Does this happen a lot? Expert: I believe so. Counsel: You are experienced in these matters. Have you ever seen it happen and could you describe it for me? Can you see anyone in this room doing this right now? Expert: Sorry, I can't. It's not something you can see. Counsel: But you are saying that it happens all the time. Have you ever seen it demonstrated by some laboratory or radiographic test? Expert: No, I haven't. Counsel: Can you demonstrate it to the Court, show us how you determine that someone is repressing something. Expert: I can't. I would have to spend time with that person. Counsel: What would you see or hear then that would be convincing to you? Expert: It would be a memory that had been lost and now re-surfaces. Counsel: Can you see or hear this as it emerges? Expert: It's a conclusion I would draw on the basis of my experience. Counsel: We have gone full circle. Please explain how the court can accept as evidence something even you, the expert can't see or hear or demonstrate in any way. Expert: (before

leaving the stand): You should give me some credit." (That's a verbatim quote from an actual x-examination.)
Here's my olive branch to the expert: Should it become possible to make visible the process of repression and denial by a radiographic method or otherwise, I will accept it. It's happened before with minimal brain injury that had been invisible in football and hockey players. Back then I doubted it. Now it seems to be beyond dispute. Maybe the same will happen with repression, although I doubt it.

Some "illnesses" seem to occur only in courtrooms, never in clinical practice. According to one claim a collapsing bed caused PTSD. According to two other claims accidents caused complete muteness in the absence of any neurological abnormality. One particularly interesting claim concerned a broken leg. The fracture was straightforward but the story that went with it was most unusual. The door to a high-rise garbage depository had been faulty. The plaintiff hadn't noticed this and found herself locked inside when she tried to leave the depository. She "had to get out of there," feeling "claustrophobic." Now to the unusual bit: With surprising determination she climbed into the narrow garbage chute, intending to slide down one floor and exit from there. But she lost her footing and careened all the way down to the ground floor into a garbage compactor. Fortunately it was turned off. She broke a leg in the process and claimed damages on grounds of claustrophobia plus managerial negligence.

Some cases can be outright entertaining, literally, like the one of **"Subway Elvis."** Elvis was a busker who performed in Toronto subway stations. He became the prime suspect after a robber held up a bank wearing an Elvis costume. Subway Elvis was convicted and did time. An alibi turned up some time later and exonerated him. The Crown ended up in the unhappy role of defending HRM and the taxpayer against a claim for wrongful conviction. Elvis had to see me for a mandatory defense medical. I expected a disgruntled plaintiff who didn't want to be there. How wrong I was. Our receptionist announced breathlessly "Elvis is here!" And there he was, in full regalia, black hair gleaming, wearing over-sized sunglasses, white imitation leather jacket and pants, two-tone boots and bells that jingled with every movement. He carried his guitar and offered to perform. Sadly, I had to carry out my boring duties and never got to hear "love me tender, love me sweet…" And I did have to "let him go." My next medico-legal was already pacing in the waiting room.

16. A Day at the Office

Years ago I visited Sigmund Freud's office at the *Berggasse* in Vienna. Books, pictures, masks and antiques gave it an aura of mystery and thoughtful contemplation. Something unique had happened there. For the first time in modern psychiatric history patients could claim the undivided attention of a doctor for hours of his time and receive his considered opinion. I admit to a nostalgic attachment to the scene. Back then psychiatrists doubled as philosophers, notably Karl Jaspers with his existentialism. Their proclivity towards careful observation and reflection is worth perpetuating. Nowadays psychiatrists are just as short of time as other medical specialists and act the harried part. Compared to the *Berggasse*, Anxiety Disorders and the Smythe Pain Clinic looked almost aseptic with their vinyl desks, filing cabinets and computers. The Smythe Pain Clinic wasn't even part of the Department of Psychiatry. It was part of Anesthesia. The pressing demand for services necessitated the strictest discipline. We had waiting lists. Schedules were planned to the minute and sometimes months in advance. Rarely did I get to know clients closely enough to remember them by name unless someone stuck out. You can't get any further away from bearded pipe-smoking psychoanalysis where a few clients spend years with their doctor.

Now to my confession: In addition to the clinics I kept a private office. It was devoted to psychotherapy with clients who could benefit from extensive intervention and to those who wouldn't be seen dead in a psychiatric facility. It was a throwback of sorts to the old days, had two large stained-glass windows, two fireplaces, Art Deco plaster and personal knick-knacks. It looked almost Freudian. And it gave me a chance to be a little less clinical and more philosophical.

I made all appointments in person. The door to the waiting room was open to the street and clients let themselves in. The arrangement had its risks, tolerable as it turned out. Only three people walked in unannounced over some thirty years. One sat on my doorstep early one morning just as I was leaving for the hospital. He was severely distressed and I was glad he had come. The other two were of a different order altogether. One made clinking noises in the waiting room. He was a lad in his twenties, a trainee burglar, nervous and almost apologetic. He pretended to be a workman. I asked for a look into his tool bag. He muttered something and left. The second intruder was a pro. He was bulky, scowled menacingly and had a prison pallor. He smashed a lock in the hope of goodies that weren't there. I approached him with caution and stepped aside as he hurried out the door and into a get-away car. Apart from this peace reigned.

It seemed strange at times to advise some very accomplished people, journalists, police officers, entrepreneurs, bankers, stockbrokers, doctors, lawyers, writers, artists, researchers and real estate agents, you name it. But they came, often just to talk. Many combined an anxiety disorder with a physical ailment, with gastro-intestinal discomfort, faintness, dizziness, breathlessness or palpitations. I used behavioral techniques and self-help literature whenever fitting, including the "One Minute Manager" by Ken Blanchard and Spencer Johnson, Claire Weekes' "Hope and Help for your Nerves" and Isaac Marks' " Living with Fear," to name just a few. Pavlov's dogs served as an introduction to classical conditioning and understanding puzzling "psychosomatic" symptoms. B.F. Skinner's "Beyond Freedom and Dignity" introduced the concept of reinforcement (or incentives as economists call it) and how this related to motivation and re-designing daily routines. Coping with stress was a common concern and how to maintain change. As Bernard Shaw put it so cogently: "It's easy to quit smoking. I have done it many times."

Motivation is the Achilles heel of psychotherapy. An old joke describes it best: "How many psychiatrists does it take to change a light bulb? – Only one. But for that the light bulb really has to want changing."

What is it that motivates people to change? According to President Bush Sr. "it's the vision thing." A need for change may be perfectly obvious to the outsider but unconvincing to the client. Such cases gave me a chance to turn philosophical. What really mattered to the client? What made sense when looking at the trajectory of her life? What barred her way towards self-fulfillment? These questions could be explored along behavioral lines: What had been the most fulfilling times in her life? What were her rewards and punishments, her incentives and disincentives then and now that motivated her? (For rewards and incentives see B.F. Skinner, alternatively Steven Levitt and Stephen Dubner in "Freakonomics" and Tim Harford in "The Undercover Economist.") Why was she here now? Did she feel depressed, hopeless and helpless, no longer expecting to turn into reality what she once hoped for? If depression was severe and came with a loss of appetite and energy plus early morning awakening, our discussion would turn to antidepressants. I would recommend but decisions had to be consensual.

It would be amiss without including my "fourth office" in the streets of Toronto. This one was different again and purely behavioral, devoted to challenging fears and phobias in the real world. A minority of clients needed and wanted this extra dose of reality. I walked crowded streets and malls with agoraphobics, rode the subway from end to end and back again and spent many hours in cars with accident survivors. I lunched on the top of high rises with height phobics and the survivors of a hotel fire, borrowed cats from friends and snakes from pet shops and sourced a supply of dead mice from the hospital lab to supplement my office equipment. In vivo exposure was a relatively small part of my practice. But it was incredibly rewarding and instructive.

One of my first clients was a bird phobic, too phobic even to know what a bird looked like close-up or how feathers felt. I acquired a mechanical bird that flapped its wings and made squawking noises. Letting it loose in St. Mike's Hospital hallways was marvelous fun but ineffective. I tried a stuffed owl and this worked better. Once my client had managed to hold the owl and stroke it we went for walks outside. She noticed birds from hundreds of meters away, even little ones. How could she tolerate getting close and personal? Would they swoop down and attack, replaying Hitchcock's movie? We studied bird behavior together and the fact that food and fear motivates them, not a desire to attack. Success was defined as her ability to feed the geese at Toronto Harbor. She mastered it and went on to visit beaches, traveled freely and proved it by sending me a postcard.

Rubber snakes made a good starter for a snake phobic. She wouldn't go anyplace with tall grass, because snakes might hide there. Tropical destinations were completely out of reach. With some encouragement she agreed to handle a rubber snake, later dead eels from Toronto's St. Lawrence Market. Eventually she felt ready to face the real thing. I rented a mid-sized python from an obliging pet shop. Unbeknownst to her I also hid a small ax under my couch before our first session with the snake. I am better now. So is she. She passed her ultimate test with a trip to a snake-ridden country in Southeast Asia. And I became friendly with the milk snake in our basement. She even has a name.

Three rules seemed wise to follow with exposure therapy: Never ask a client to do something you might not be prepared to do yourself. Never ever spring a surprise like "voila here's the mouse." Let the client approach the feared situation at her own pace, even if it takes hours. Don't shove it at even the bravest client. And, most importantly, never fail to confront fear without interruption once you started. Keep it up for as long as it takes to extinguish the urge to leave (or you will make matters worse). Fight must win out over flight. Homework practice is needed afterwards to make improvement stick. Repeated practice under varying conditions, first in the presence, then in the absence of the therapist is vital before "graduation."

I used slides as supplement, of heights, planes and certain sexual matters, projected onto a wide screen to make it look as real as possible. The CBC kindly provided soundtracks of thunderstorms and incoming artillery fire to help with unusual phobias. These mock-ups were only a pale preview of what's possible now with the help of virtual reality. Recently at the MASSMOCA museum I sat comfortably in an easy chair wearing a headset while flying high over New York. The trip included a few special treats. My plane disintegrated in flight while I continued through space with nothing but my virtual seat and New York beneath. Debris and floating typewriters provided the in-flight entertainment. Virtual reality setups like this one may cost real money. But they are cheap, considering their potential benefits. Taking agoraphobics on virtual walks, flight phobics on virtual plane rides and social phobics into virtual meetings will be more powerful than imaginary exposure and far less cumbersome than arranging in-vivo exposure (meeting the real thing). It will save therapist time and increase access to treatment.

This much about therapy. What about the therapist?" A cartoon from Punch magazine portrays a wise man with a long straggly beard. He sits cross-legged on a rocky cliff, beneath him his disciple, looking equally haggard. The disciple implores: "Master, how can you keep so calm?" "Well," speaks the master, "I scream a lot." I also coped by getting away from work as far as I could in my spare time and never ever "analyzed everything said in conversation" as some suggest for my pastime. At work I did my level best to never cross one very important red line: My personal agenda must not supersede my client's. She decides what her priorities are, not me. It's easy to disappoint though and in ways one wouldn't expect.

Once a man asked for me by name at the clinic. I obliged and we had our talk. First he seemed satisfied. But then, on his way out the door he turned and asked: "Are you really Dr. Kuch?" Puzzled, I replied in the affirmative, pointing to my nametag. He was unconvinced. "Well," he said, "you are ok. But I really wanted to see the Pakistani doctor." "A Pakistani psychiatrist by the same name?" I had to check. A second look at his chart reassured me that I had indeed seen him before. But this was in the summer. Now it was winter and I no longer matched the tanned looks of "the Pakistani doctor."

It's also possible to disappoint on the upside. Once upon a time I was the proud owner of a second-hand Chevy Impala '64 convertible, the beloved one from Florida. It was black with a wide ragtop and sported red leather seats that were as wide as a sofa. It had eaten a few miles and lived through "a few wars," as one grease monkey put it. I had longish hair then and a Zapata moustache. A long summer weekend was ending and I was on my way back to Toronto, driving along happily, top down, wind in my hair and looking a little worse for wear. A police cruiser pulled up and stayed in the lane besides me. I continued to drive along while religiously observing the speed limit. He thumbed me over. Dutifully, I stopped. He got out of his cruiser and ordered me out as well. I complied. He said: "Walk around the car." I did, and steadily. He studied my "MD" license plates (issued then to licensed Ontario physicians), demanded to see my papers and a second ID. He took his time studying these. Still incredulous he asked: "Are you a doctor?" I assured him I was. He gave me a long thoughtful look, then turned to his partner in the cruiser. "I guess it must be true" he said. And with that they drove off.

17. Before I Go

Fourteen years ago I retired in stages and with regret. The Pain Clinic got the chop first, then Anxiety Disorders and the private office. Forensics and a mood disorders clinic at the Royal Victoria Hospital in Barrie came last. Many sad good-byes happened on the way. My "failures" had stayed with me for years. They knew little about me personally but there was a bond. I was walking away from people who had depended on me. I called in old favors to refer them elsewhere; but it felt sad.

One old-timer took a cutting from an office plant as a memento. Others were tearful. A few traveled almost a hundred miles to the clinic at the Royal Victoria Hospital to continue seeing me during my last two years of practice. And then I took my seat "in God's waiting room" as Ray Evans used to call it. All of a sudden I had time on my hands, time for memories and time for thoughts about death and dying.

And then I realized that this was another chance for a tilt at the windmills.

My father died from a heart attack when he was only 55 years old. His first heart attack struck him in the middle of a November night. An ambulance took him to the hospital where he worked. I was at his bedside within hours and spent the next week there, hunched over textbooks and studying for my medical boards. The window of his hospital room looked out over the river and the hills where we had spent so much time together. He described the pain he had felt in his chest during that fateful night, "sharp and severe like severing a finger." He was determined to recover and looked forward to the woods and the river. His condition stabilized. I returned to Heidelberg to focus on my studies. I had been there for only a few days when a telegram arrived at the student residence. My dad had suffered a second infarct. A strange sense of detachment took over as I gathered up essential study materials and left Heidelberg, speeding through evening gloom and rain. Ominously, an elevator waited for me at the ground floor of the hospital with its doors open. He was in the same room as before. Pillows supported his neck and head, keeping him half upright to ease his labored breathing. An IV was running. Oxygen-conducting tubes were in his nose. He was agitated and claustrophobic and fought off an oxygen tent. He had been giving last instructions to my step-mom until breathlessness and confusion took over. I held his hand, felt his racing pulse and looked into his terrified eyes. He struggled and shifted, seemingly unable to recognize me. Hours passed. His pulse grew fainter and ever more irregular, his breathing increasingly strained. His agony continued until close to midnight when his doctor told us that all hope was lost. He rapidly pushed the contents of a syringe into a vein. My father's lips moved a few more times, mimicking breath. Then came the hiss of oxygen being disconnected and silence. I had witnessed an assisted death.

Another experience made me think again about assisted death, this one decades later and very different. I was assessing an elderly lady in a large nursing home in regards to a compensation claim. The staff were exceptionally kind, the building spacious and clean. And it horrified me. The large entrance hall was well lit by a glass dome overhead but lacked a view to the outside. Some twenty inmates sat there, slumped in wheelchairs that had been arranged in a semi-circle. An eerie silence reigned as their eyes followed me. Boredom was palpable. I was the event of the day. I found my client in her bed in a room with curtains drawn. She clutched a life-size doll, disoriented and terrified by my intrusion. The doll was her only consolation, regardless of staff's efforts to reassure her. Her condition was chronic but not life threatening. It condemned her to wait until death released her.

I was visiting my own personal nightmare.

Both my dad and the above-mentioned lady didn't have a choice. In a sad way dad was lucky. His doctor took pity on him and saved him from slow asphyxiation by pulmonary edema, if only at the last minute. The old lady was just as helpless but without relief. She'd be either bored silly or terrified and confused, if still alive. I knew others who endured their last years in similar ways while wishing they were dead. And these were the ones who were getting decent care. I hate to think of the others. Which gets me to Dying With Dignity (DwD), a charitable organization with sister organizations in many countries and more that a few battles for medical assistance in dying (MAID) under its belt. I hope that my doctor will save me from a lengthy agony and from ending up helpless and bored silly in a nursing home. I am putting this request into my Advance Care Directive.

The Western world decriminalized suicide many decades ago as part of a larger trend that has given people more rights over their body. Pain relief has obtained priority over prolonging life (according to WHO guidelines for palliative care). The administration of large doses of potent pain relievers is now acceptable even when it (accidentally) hastens death. Switzerland, Belgium and the Netherlands went further and decriminalized MAID, followed by a growing number of US States and Canada. The battle isn't over yet. It continues to rage over rules and limits. What I would like to know is how, in a continent where "minding your own business" is a stock phrase, religious and administrative interference continues to limit personal choice even when no harm will result from it. Yet common sense is uncommon when it comes to an issue as emotionally charged as MAID. The current Canadian legislation still has gaps. To someone with progressive dementia the restriction of MAID to a "foreseeable" death offers a Hobson's choice: Go to Switzerland for a needlessly early death or wait and endure until loss of competence bars you from travel and MAID. Canadian Law also does not address the requests of "mature minors," children who are capable of understanding the implications of their request while not meeting age requirements. And it does not address intolerable suffering that is beyond remediation in competent persons with a mental illness.

We strive to improve quality of life. We should strive to improve quality of death as well.

I am not in a hurry though.

How does one outfox the prospect of it all ending in one huge downer? That's not the way to end a book or a life. To put the question more positively, how does one maintain quality of life right up to the end? I plan to have fun the way I always had until the music stops, with as few concessions to age as possible. I expect to tilt at a few more windmills and argue the case for objective thought for as long as I can, in medicine and in politics. I want to champion openness, mutual support beyond borders and the mobility of talent. They should be available to others as they were to me, so they too can find their place.

Over to you.

18. About The Author

Klaus Kuch is a retired associate professor of psychiatry with a cross-appointment in anesthesia. Initially he worked full-time, later part-time at the University of Toronto. His special interests include behavioral and cognitive therapy, anxiety, depression pain and forensics. He has published some 60 related scientific articles and book chapters.

He went to medical school in Germany and qualified as a general practitioner there, later also in Canada. For his psychiatric specialty training he moved to the University of Florida in Gainesville and later to Toronto, qualifying in the US and Canada as a specialist.

In Toronto he practiced at the University Health Network, first at St. Michael's Hospital, then at Toronto General Hospital, at the Center of Addiction and Mental Health and later at the Royal Victoria Hospital in Barrie, Ontario. He consulted for the Consulate General of Germany, the Ontario Workplace Safety and Insurance Board (WSIB) and its Appeals Tribunal. He provided medico-legal assessments for the Ontario College of Physicians and Surgeons, the Crown Law Office and numerous law firms in civil and criminal litigation cases.

He lives on a farm, is married, intermittently interested in sports and consistently interested in fun. He keeps chickens occasionally but refuses to have anything to do with cattle.

The author may be reached at https://www.linkedin.com/
Email oldbones345@bell.net
Most of his research publications can be found on www.researchgate.net

Made in the USA
Monee, IL
20 January 2020